Praying Through Infertility

a 90-day devotional
for men & women

Praying Through Infertility

*a 90-day devotional
for men & women*

COMPILED BY

SHERIDAN VOYSEY

W PUBLISHING GROUP

AN IMPRINT OF THOMAS NELSON

Published in Nashville, Tennessee, by W Publishing, an imprint of Thomas Nelson.

Thomas Nelson titles may be purchased in bulk for educational, business, fundraising, or sales promotional use. For information, please email SpecialMarkets@ThomasNelson.com.

Unless otherwise noted, Scripture quotations are taken from the Holy Bible, New International Version®, NIV®. Copyright © 1973, 1978, 1984, 2011 by Biblica, Inc.® Used by permission of Zondervan. All rights reserved worldwide. www.zondervan.com. The "NIV" and "New International Version" are trademarks registered in the United States Patent and Trademark Office by Biblica, Inc.®

Scripture quotations marked CEV are taken from the Contemporary English Version. Copyright © 1991, 1992, 1995 by American Bible Society. Used by permission.

Scripture quotations marked ESV are taken from the ESV® Bible (The Holy Bible, English Standard Version®). Copyright © 2001 by Crossway, a publishing ministry of Good News Publishers. Used by permission. All rights reserved.

Scripture quotations marked MSG are taken from THE MESSAGE. Copyright © 1993, 2002, 2018 by Eugene H. Peterson. Used by permission of NavPress. All rights reserved. Represented by Tyndale House Publishers, a Division of Tyndale House Ministries.

Scripture quotations marked NKJV are taken from the New King James Version®. Copyright © 1982 by Thomas Nelson. Used by permission. All rights reserved.

Scripture quotations marked NLT are taken from the Holy Bible, New Living Translation. Copyright © 1996, 2004, 2015 by Tyndale House Foundation. Used by permission of Tyndale House Ministries, Carol Stream, Illinois 60188. All rights reserved.

Scripture quotations marked NLV are taken from the New Life Version. © 1969, 2003 by Barbour Publishing, Inc.

Scripture quotations marked TLB are taken from The Living Bible. Copyright © 1971. Used by permission of Tyndale House Publishers, a Division of Tyndale House Ministries, Carol Stream, Illinois 60188. All rights reserved.

ISBN 978-1-4003-3453-7 (audiobook)
ISBN 978-1-4003-3452-0 (eBook)
ISBN 978-1-4003-3451-3 (softcover)

Library of Congress Control Number: 2023937374

Printed in the United States of America
23 24 25 26 27 LBC 5 4 3 2 1

Contents

Contents

Contents

Contents

You Are Not Alone

—— Introduction ——

The memory is vivid: the doctor sitting there quietly, his hands clasped and resting on the desk while my wife stares vacantly at a lamp in the corner and I search the floor for something to say. The doctor's few words have somehow bled the color from the room. Like a desaturated photo, all around us is now gray—gray walls, gray chairs, gray papers, pens, plants, hearts.

"What about IVF?" Merryn says, pulling a tissue from her handbag, her chin beginning to quiver.

The doctor watches my wife for a moment, assessing her readiness for more disappointment, then glances at the file in front of him. "With these results, regular IVF won't be any help to you," he says. "The sperm count is just too low."

"So that's it?" I say, guilty feelings already forming at being the cause of the problem, feelings that will take years to shift.

"No," the doctor replies, "there's one medical option open to you—ICSI, or intracytoplasmic sperm injection. It's a form of IVF where a single sperm is injected into an egg in the lab to help it fertilize, and the resulting embryo is then transferred into the uterus."

We fall silent for a while, trying to make sense of what we're hearing, reality slowly dawning that what is so easily achieved for others will be difficult for us.

"There's always adoption," the doctor adds. "And, of course, some couples in your situation just choose to remain childless."

We leave the gray office, step into a gray street and toward our gray car—the first steps of a journey we'd never chosen. And of all that we'd face in the coming years, one of the hardest feelings felt would be that of loneliness.

———————————

To have come to hold a book like this, you may have had a similar experience to what I've shared or are in the nebulous early stage of waiting for answers. While the details of our experiences will differ, the emotions probably won't. You've felt the same growing sense of worry as conception hasn't happened, maybe the same shock and sadness we experienced if a diagnosis has been given, the same sense of unfairness at being singled out for this, perhaps the same confusion over the options you now have to assess, and maybe a little fear about making a wrong decision. Like us, you may have felt some loneliness too—that no one around you really understands. Infertility isn't a typical topic of café conversation. It can take years to meet others who've experienced it, and so couples like us can easily feel isolated.

Introduction

Praying Through Infertility was written to let you know that you are in fact *not* alone:

- not alone in your sadness, anger, or confusion;
- not alone when you feel jealous of parents who have what you want;
- not alone when a giggling child brings not delight but grief;
- not alone in wondering who you'll be if you never become a mother or father.

You are not alone if you've had to concoct a clever excuse to avoid a baby shower, or if a friend's pregnancy announcement has left you in tears, or if you can't face another Mother's or Father's Day at church. You are not alone if looking into in vitro fertilization (IVF), donor eggs or sperm, the adoption process, or other family-building options leaves you bewildered, or if differing opinions about moving forward have raised tensions in your marriage. And you are not alone if all this has pulled at the threads of your faith, fraying your relationship with God as you've wondered why He hasn't yet done for you what He did for the Sarahs, Hannahs, and Elizabeths of Scripture, or the others you know whose prayers seemingly brought forth a miracle baby.

Although it took a while to discover, what Merryn and I didn't know back in that doctor's office was that there was a hidden tribe of people who *did* understand this experience with every fiber of their being—a tribe with members not just across the globe but also in our cities and churches, who'd been through the wilderness of infertility, had the scars to prove it, and could be helpful guides to the terrain.

No, you are not alone in this experience called *infertility*. A tribe of fellow journeyers exists, and God Himself is walking by your side.

I remember the day I first met another tribe member. It happened a year or so after that fateful doctor's appointment—our fertility journey not having moved much beyond some "fertility-boosting" diets while I wrestled with the ethics of technologies like ICSI. Passing a café one day, I was beckoned by someone I knew to join him and his friends inside. How the conversation began I don't recall, and neither do I remember his name, but soon I was telling the man sitting next to me about Merryn's and my infertility. He replied that he and his wife had done IVF twice, and my relief at finding someone who *knew* the ordeal was palpable.

In the years ahead Merryn and I would try numerous rounds of ICSI treatment, more diets and special supplements, chiropractic consults (I have no idea why), and healing prayer. We would endure a year of intrusive assessment as potential adoptive parents before embarking on a two-year wait for a hoped-for adoptive child. While we had caring companions along the way, it was still difficult to meet other tribe members.

Our turning point in finding them finally came by going public with our story.

This was no small move. While I had spoken professionally for years, I'd never mentioned our fertility struggle—both of us were content to keep it private. But prompted by a friend, we shared our experience in a book called *Resurrection Year* and in a follow-up title called *The Making of Us*. The result was an overflowing inbox for several years, with readers from around the world telling us their own stories. Men confided to us their sense of shame over not being able to father a child. Women shared their crises of purpose, wondering who they'd be without motherhood. Broken marriages, lost faith, even emotional breakdowns—we heard the deepest heartbreaks, many never shared before. Going public with our story seemed to permit others to share their own.

And then wonderful things started to happen. As the secret griefs came into the light, as stories were heard and prayers prayed, shame began to lift, marriages started to mend, faith was renewed, and new purpose found. It was not all at once, and not without further difficulty. But like my meeting with the stranger in the café, finding other members of the tribe led to burdens being shared as God recycled our wilderness experiences into redemptive help for each other.

Our prayer is that you'll find such comradery, too, and we're confident you won't have long to wait. Why? Because *Praying Through Infertility* was written by those we've met along the path, people who've been where you are now.

Introduction

People like:

- David and Lizzie, who've learned through their ordeal how to be more emotionally healthy and how grieving well can be a path back to joy;
- Tim and Dorcas, who found powerful ways to strengthen their marriage when infertility was pulling them apart;
- Sheila, who knows how to respond graciously but honestly to a friend's pregnancy news, and Katherine, who's learned not to put life on hold while waiting;
- plus Sarah and Steph, who remind us of how playlists and pets can bring moments of levity on the journey, and Rômulo, Lori, Claire, and Sikhumbuzo, who've found that praying even through their deep disappointments has expanded their visions of God.

There are nearly forty of us ready to greet you in these pages. Come and meet us as if we were waiting for you in that café. We are American, Australian, British, Brazilian, Canadian, Filipino, Romanian, Singaporean, and Zimbabwean, with different outcomes to our journeys. Some of us have been blessed with biological children, some have formed families through fostering or adoption, others are walking forward childless, and a few are still on the path. We come from a variety of denominations and have experienced between us many of the medical options available, from IVF to donor eggs and sperm. What we share is an experience of infertility's dark depths and a faith that's held strong through the testing.

We've been praying for you and have some things to share that might help in the days ahead. So come, take a seat. Let us help ease the load.

———————————

Off the northwest coast of Italy is a small cove accessible only by boat or on foot. Walking through the wilderness to reach it, you find a secluded abbey on its slopes and an even greater surprise in its bay. As you wade into the cove and sink deeper and deeper into its dark waters, two raised hands come into view. This is *Christ of the Abyss*, the world's first underwater statue, placed in 1954. Jesus stands on the sea floor, His hands raised to heaven, ready to meet those in the depths.[1]

The depths. Infertility can feel like that—dark and overwhelming in its griefs. And just as He met Mary Magdalene in the depths of sadness on Easter morning, and Peter in the depths of shame after denying Him three times, and Cleopas in the depths of confusion as He walked the Emmaus road, Jesus is ready to meet us in our shadowy waters. The One who left the brilliance of heaven for earth's dark streets has always specialized in meeting us in the depths and lifting us out in time.

This book isn't about talking through or empathizing with infertility alone. We don't just have guidance to offer but prayers—prayers that can become yours when your own words fail, prayers that can lead you up for breath. Each entry you read

Introduction

in this ninety-day devotional is grounded in Scripture, where transformative power resides, and crafted to facilitate prayer, where real change happens. Forasmuch as infertility can have us wondering why God at times seems silent, there is no one better than Him to guide us on this path, let alone transform its sufferings into growth and purpose. "I will exalt you, LORD, for you lifted me out of the depths" (Psalm 30:1). Those raised arms are raised for us. There is resurrection power in those hands.

Praying Through Infertility was written for you to read together as a couple, but we know there are times when one partner just isn't ready to join in. You might like to find a caring friend to read with you instead, or just engage personally. A prompt has been included at the end of each entry to help you reflect on its theme. Journaling your thoughts and prayers in response can be a powerful way to meet God through each entry. It can be helpful, too, to sit prayerfully with each day's theme—rather than reading ahead—letting it do its work in you.

As you read and as you pray, may peace, hope, and trust meet you this day.

He is with us. And we are with you.

You are not alone.

SHERIDAN VOYSEY

Riding the Roller Coaster

*The light shines in the darkness, and
the darkness has not overcome it.*

I liken our infertility journey to a roller-coaster ride. Every month we'd start out with hope—perhaps *this* would be the month. Then we'd have the anxious two-week wait after ovulation before the crushing disappointment that the onset of my period would bring.

I am not a fan of roller coasters. If you can persuade me onto one at all, I'll have my eyes tightly closed through the stomach-losing drops and scary parts. It's tempting to do the same when it comes to the challenging emotions that accompany infertility. No one likes feeling anxious, fearful, or disappointed. Added to this, as followers of Jesus, we can experience a sense of shame for feeling as we do. If we trust God, we surely shouldn't feel anxious or fearful, right?

I have always loved the opening of John's gospel. It speaks to the beautiful truth that God, through the person of Jesus, didn't expect us to find our own way out of darkness; instead, Jesus meets us in our darkness. Jesus entered all the brokenness and pain of this world, and rather than being consumed by the dark, He lit it up with His love (John 1:1–5).

Rather than trying to deny how we feel, we can invite Jesus into the darkness of our emotions. We can talk with Him openly and honestly about how we feel. I can't say I managed to do this every time I felt anxious or disappointed during our walk with infertility, but when I did, I experienced the comfort of His loving presence. It was the presence of Jesus that lit up my darkness.

Thank You, Jesus, that You enter into our darkness. Today I'm feeling [insert your own emotion here]. Help me to experience Your loving presence in this place. Thank You that Your love illuminates my darkness. Amen.

KATHERINE GANTLETT

Invite Jesus to bring His light into your anxiety, fear, and disappointment.

Dealing with Diagnosis

———————— 2 ————————

This child is destined to cause the falling
and rising of many in Israel, and to be a
sign that will be spoken against.

LUKE 2:22–40

Four words sent my world tumbling down: "You have zero sperm."

With those four words I received my infertility diagnosis, and with it my identity, masculinity, and faith received a gut punch. Something I'd never questioned—my capacity to father children—was suddenly and shockingly out of reach. That day in the waiting room, I was left googling "azoospermia," frantically figuring out what medical options were available. Within a few months the pressure of dealing with my diagnosis spiraled into a mental health breakdown that would take months to recover from. Life after those four words was irreversibly different.

How do we deal with bad news? What reservoirs of faith can fill the emptiness such gut punches bring?

Six weeks after their angels-and-shepherds moment, Mary and Joseph presented their baby in the temple (Luke 2:22). There Simeon blessed them but said that their child would cause the "falling and rising of many" (v. 34). Bad news! Even more, Mary was told that because of Jesus, "a sword will pierce your own soul too" (v. 35). We're not told Mary's response at this point, but at the end of Luke 2, we read she "treasured all these things in her heart" (v. 51).

Looking back, I can see that the bad news of my diagnosis became like a brick wall around my heart. I was numb, afraid, and lacked Mary's courage to open my heart and ultimately trust God with my pain. When I finally did, I found the deep and knowing love of God, whose diagnosis went beyond "You have no sperm" to "You are 'fearfully and wonderfully made'" (Psalm 139:14). Trusting God with my diagnosis, and my heart, helped to ease the pain.

God of love, when bad news comes, help me to open my heart so I can know Your presence in the midst of pain and hold on to Your truth about who I am. May I not become hard-hearted but have the heart of Mary, who was able to trust You even when her whole life changed. Amen.

ELIS MATTHEWS

Placing your diagnosis into God's hands can keep your heart soft toward Him and each other.

The Opportunity
of Exile

———— 3 ————

*You will seek me and find me when
you seek me with all your heart.*

JEREMIAH 29:10–14

T he doctor's diagnosis of unexplained infertility plummeted me into a pit of despair. What shape would our lives take if we never had children? How long would we have to wait to know if we definitely wouldn't? The diagnosis felt like an exile to an unknown land without any idea when or if we'd ever leave.

The Jews encountered exile; it was uninvited, and a long wait ensued until they returned home and rebuilt their lives (Jeremiah 30:3). Yet in the midst of this unsettled time, the exile provided fertile ground for God to reveal His plans for them. He hadn't abandoned them but longed for them to use that time to seek Him in their waiting, coming to know Him better (29:13).

I discovered this to be true of my own exile. Since waiting solely for a pregnancy produced little else but disappointment in me, I accepted God's invitation to discover Him more during this time of waiting. I devoted entire mornings to reading His Word, praying, and journaling, and found myself immersed in His lovely dwelling place (Psalm 84:1). Investing time with God brought a renewing of my mind (Romans 12:2) and peace to my soul. What started as an unwelcome medical diagnosis resulted in an opportunity to discover God's incredible capacity to sustain me and the revelation that His grace is sufficient for me (2 Corinthians 12:9).

Infertility can feel like an exile to an unknown land, fueling uncertainty around when and if we'll ever leave. But God wants to reveal something more about Himself to you in this time. Seek Him and He will meet you.

Lord, waiting for pregnancy is hard, and not knowing when it will happen is even harder. As I wait, please grow in me the desire to know You better. Amen.

AMANDA PICKERING

How can you turn this time of waiting into a time of waiting on God, ready to receive what He wishes to reveal?

He Knows You

---------- 4 ----------

You know when I sit down or stand up.
You know my thoughts even when I'm far away.
PSALM 139:1–16 NLT

He knows you. He knows every detail and nanosecond of your existence—every atom, molecule, skin cell, and ligament, every hope, dream, sadness, and achievement. He knows you intimately, through and through.

He knows every movement you will make today (Psalm 139:2–3)—every action, step, and pause for rest, every blink, glance, and breath. He knows each thought you will have—every joy, question, and concern—and every word you will speak before you speak them (v. 4). He knows your complete personality—your emotional triggers, behavioral patterns, bad habits, and comfort zones. He knows what you're good at, bad at, tempted by, and victorious over. He can unravel the intricate workings of your heart when you remain confused.

There is no rock large enough, no place far enough, no darkness thick enough to hide you from Him (vv. 7–12). He was there as you were crafted in the womb (vv. 13–15) and knows the events to take place on your final day on earth (v. 16). He knows what your future holds and the paths you'll take to get there. Because He knows you.

This is good news for us because infertility can leave us feeling unseen and unknown. Few around us have faced its griefs, fewer still seem able to empathize, and sometimes we lack the words for all we're experiencing, leaving us unknown even to ourselves. But the objective fact beyond all feelings to the contrary, the truth as true as the sun's existence at nighttime, is this: He knows everything about you, and He knows it thoroughly. Even, and especially, this.

Lord, when others don't get it and even I am confused, You know all that I'm experiencing and understand my life perfectly. Thank You for attending to my life in such intimate detail and being trustworthy of all it holds. Amen.

SHERIDAN VOYSEY

There is no detail of your journey He doesn't know.

A Gracious Alliance

———————— 5 ————————

A cord of three strands is not quickly broken.
ECCLESIASTES 4:9–12

When sexual dysfunction and infertility holed our marriage below the waterline, my wife, Dorcas, and I didn't man the pumps or really attempt to fix the damage; we just unconsciously climbed into separate life rafts and drifted apart. We were being tossed around by the same waves, but our experiences and emotions were radically different. Dorcas was drowning in grief and a sense of abandonment, while I was crippled by fear and shame. But because of our emotional distance, we couldn't understand what the other was going through, which made the hurt and frustration worse. Emotionally we were like the person the writer of Ecclesiastes pitied, who "falls and has no one to help them up" (4:10).

When intrauterine insemination enabled us to conceive for the first and only time, our hopes soared. But our marriage had taken on too much water and practically went under when we had a miscarriage. Thankfully, around this time the Lord brought across our path an excellent biblical counselor, who encouraged us to form a "gracious alliance" in our grief and shame. That advice was a marriage saver for us, starting us down the path of becoming the kind of couple that helps each other up when we fall (vv. 9–10).

One afternoon, Dorcas and I walked and talked for hours, trying to understand how the other was feeling and experiencing our struggle. Dorcas told me she felt abandoned, and I told her I felt ashamed. We committed before the Lord to be open and honest, bringing everything out into the light. This meant humbling ourselves and being vulnerable as we asked for help from each other and the Lord.

It takes no effort to drift apart in a marriage, but it takes true strength to face a painful trial like infertility together in a gracious alliance. Now a three-strand cord has been woven that binds us together with the Lord. It won't be easily broken (v. 12).

Father, be that third strand in my marriage as I seek to understand my spouse and how they're experiencing our infertility. Help me to prove two are better than one, that mutual vulnerability and care is a blessing You provide and enable by Your grace. May we live in closeness with each other and with You. Amen.

TIM BERRY

How can you form your own gracious alliance together?

In His Hands

We wait in hope for the LORD; he is our help and our shield.
In him our hearts rejoice, for we trust in his holy name.

PSALM 33:20–22

We were supposed to begin our next fertility cycle. But in an unexpected turn, I was now being scheduled for breast biopsies. Halted from our efforts to conceive, I pleaded with God, "No. Please, all I want is a baby." Reeling from shock and disbelief, I filled the pages of my journal with words of heartache and anger. Yet, in the Lord's loving-kindness, He revealed Psalm 33:20–22 in response to my anguish.

Psalm 33 is a song of praise describing who God is. He is trustworthy (vv. 4–5), the great Creator (vv. 6–9), full of unfailing love (v. 18), and the deliverer from death (v. 19). By declaring God's character, the psalmist encouraged the reader to praise the Lord and trust in His name. Here we see that praising God and trusting God are intertwined. When we know how good God is, we can trust Him to do what's right.

Although I was nowhere near ready to praise God in the face of my roadblock, God knew what my heart needed. In the lowest points of my infertility, He revealed the conclusion to my begging and longing. Even though I saw a split path of either fighting for my life or having a baby, God whispered from the Psalms, *Do you trust Me?*

And He was trustworthy. On the morning of my breast biopsies, I ovulated for the first time on my own, and two weeks later, the biopsies came back clear and our journey to parenthood began. Through it all the message of praising God and trusting Him was key to our waiting in hope for the Lord. In His hands, your now and your future are secure.

> *Lord, provide Your comfort, nearness, and help in my questioning. When it's hard to trust You, Lord, may I know that You are the only One who can hold me in the waiting, the unknowns, and the roadblocks. Guide my heart to Your truth, Your will, and Your story for my life over my own. Lord, help me to love You for who You are, not just what You can give me.*

> KELLEY RAMSEY

In His hands, your now and your future are secure.

Waiting in Trust

———— 7 ————

Overhearing what they said, Jesus told him,
"Don't be afraid; just believe."

MARK 5:21–43

It took us several years to conceive our daughter, Laura, who finally came to us with the help of IVF treatment. During those years of waiting, we were astonished at how many of our friends got pregnant unexpectedly. It wasn't always easy news for us to hear.

One day while reading the Gospel of Mark, we were struck by the story of Jairus, a father desperate for a miracle who threw himself at Jesus' feet, pleading for his daughter's healing (Mark 5:21–43). Jesus listened to Jairus and went with him, but on the way He stopped to heal a sick woman and even talk with her (vv. 24–34). This delay was long enough for Jairus's daughter to pass away, but Jesus told Jairus, "Don't be afraid; just believe" (vv. 35–36). Believe in what? Jesus didn't say He would heal the girl. All He had promised so far was His presence.

For the honor and glory of God, the healing took place (vv. 41–42). But if it hadn't, Jesus would have still been present. This story taught us to turn our problem over to Jesus, trusting that He would be with us no matter the outcome.

Praying Through Infertility

God is at work in our times of waiting, working miracles for others and preparing the outcome to our prayers. And He is present in those times when everything seems to be going wrong. Today may we cling to His words, "Don't be afraid; just believe."

Father God, may our trust in You grow stronger and stronger, knowing that You are sovereign and can do whatever You want. Help me to trust that Your presence will be enough in my life, no matter what happens. May Your mighty name be glorified in everything. Amen.

RÔMULO CORRÊA

_____

God is at work during your times of waiting.

Strength to Carry On

8

I lie down and sleep; I wake again,
because the LORD sustains me.

PSALM 3:1–8

My husband, Francisco, and I never imagined we would walk through the doors of an infertility center. With each step we took, we felt weaker and weaker. It seemed all our hopes of having a child were coming to a halt. Uncertainty, fear, and a glimmer of hope mingled in our hearts as we prepared to meet the doctor. We wondered whether we'd have the strength to carry on if faced with our worst fears.

In Psalm 3 we find King David wrestling with a grim reality he never imagined he'd face—fleeing from his own son Absalom who was trying to overthrow him from the throne. Many around David predicted a hopeless ending (v. 2), yet instead of giving in to fear, David did something unexpected. He burst into praise, singing, "But you, LORD, are a shield around me, my glory, the One who lifts my head high" (v. 3). David found strength in the Lord to carry on, knowing that he could sleep peacefully because the Lord was sustaining him (v. 5).

Leaving the fertility center that day, Francisco and I decided to focus on praising God, proclaiming His character and love for us, no matter what the ending would be. While we were finally blessed with our daughter, Esmeralda, the lesson of praising God in the middle of difficulty has never left us.

Sometimes, in a journey like this, uncertainties and fears seem almost impossible to overcome. Like David, let's find strength by proclaiming the character of God. He is our shield, the One who will sustain us.

Lord, there are days when I feel I don't have the strength to carry on anymore. Today I choose to push against my uncertainties and fears. Today I proclaim that You are my shield, the One who lifts my head high. Today I will rest because You sustain me. Today I will trust in You. Amen.

ESTERA PIROSCA ESCOBAR

What characteristic of God can you praise and hold on to today?

Glory-Based Decisions

9

*So whether you eat or drink or whatever
you do, do it all for the glory of God.*

1 CORINTHIANS 10:27–31

You have three embryos that are very poor quality," the doctor said. "For the best chance at a pregnancy, we should transfer all three to your uterus. It probably won't result in a pregnancy, but if it does, you might have triplets, which could be dangerous. If you don't transfer them, you'll have to start the process all over again, which will cost several thousand dollars more. Let us know your decision in fifteen minutes."

The difficult decision Tom and I faced that day in the fertility clinic was not unique to us. Every couple experiencing infertility faces myriad choices. *Should we adopt or foster? Should we pursue treatment or pray for a miraculous, natural conception? Is it okay to stop trying and do life without children?* Even after reading Scripture, praying, and seeking wise counsel, the answer isn't always clear.

The Bible doesn't give us specific answers to every situation, but 1 Corinthians 10:31 does give us a standard to uphold when making decisions. Paul was talking to the church in Corinth about whether they should consume food or drink sacrificed to idols (vv. 27–30). But the phrase "whatever you do" seems to imply that all our actions should be done with an effort to glorify God. We can look at every decision through the lens of this verse, using it as a guiding principle.

Infertility forces us to make many tough choices. It is easy to feel overwhelmed by the ramifications of each one. Making God's glory the basis and goal for each decision we make can help us choose well and find solace.

Lord, we want to glorify You with the decisions we make during this season of infertility. Whether You call us to adopt, to give birth to children, or to live child-free, help us to do it in a manner pleasing to You. No matter the outcome of our story, may You be glorified.

LISA NEWTON

How could a decision you currently face reveal
God's reality and goodness to the world?

Staying in Step

*That is why a man leaves his father and mother and
is united to his wife, and they become one flesh.*

GENESIS 2:18–24

I don't know whether they do it anymore, but along with egg-and-spoon races, the three-legged race was a permanent fixture of sports day when I was growing up. It was one of the few events where to complete the course, let alone win, you had to work with another person.

Infertility brings with it many difficult decisions about assisted reproductive technologies and other family-building options, which can leave you feeling like you need to become an expert in ethics and other topics just to understand the issues, let alone decide. When you add in the powerful emotions swirling around the situation, discerning how to move forward becomes a significant challenge.

Right at the beginning of the Bible, we're told in marriage two people are united to become one flesh (Genesis 2:24). Just like in a three-legged race, being united together in marriage means that we have to move at the same pace as our partner. For Jon and me, this meant we agreed not to move forward with decisions until we were united in agreement.

It was hard at times, when one of us desperately wanted

to move in a particular direction. It took a lot of trust that we were both working to discern what God wanted us to do and acting out of love and in each other's best interests. We didn't always manage it well. But I am convinced that this strategy was one of the reasons our marriage was stronger than ever at the end of our infertility journey.

Heavenly Father, thank You for the gift of marriage. Just as You encourage us to walk in step with your Spirit, help us to walk in step with each other. Help us to love well, preferring the other, and trusting that You are guiding us through it all. Amen.

KATHERINE GANTLETT

Staying in step with each other will help keep you united.

A Legacy and a Name

Let no eunuch complain,
"I am only a dry tree." . . .
To them I will give . . .
a memorial and a name
better than sons and daughters.

ISAIAH 56:3–5

For me the tinges of pain come at the most unexpected moments—hearing a little boy call out "Dad" as he plays football in the park with his father or watching a parent sitting in front of me at church attend to her wriggly child.

It's amazing that in the Old Testament God didn't overlook the pain of the childless. In Isaiah 56 He spoke directly to childless eunuchs who felt they were nothing more than "dry trees" and gave them a promise (v. 3). Historically, these eunuchs weren't considered worthy of being part of the Jewish people, and yet here they were welcomed into God's eternal kingdom. Since they "'choose what pleases me'" (v. 4), God gave them the promise of a legacy "'better than sons and daughters'" and a name that will "'endure forever'" (v. 5).

Society and church life often revolve around children. Those without can sometimes be left feeling like outcasts, much like these eunuchs of old. It's so easy to feel weighed down by our deep longings to be parents—to be that dad pushing his daughter on the swings, or that mother teaching her son to read—and too often our pain isn't acknowledged or understood. Yet God not only understands this pain, He addresses and welcomes the childless into His glorious kingdom.

What an amazing encouragement for childless Christians like me! And maybe this can encourage you, too, as you walk forward. Whatever your future, whether you have children or not, God gives you a legacy, a name, and a place in His eternal kingdom. This extravagant promise starts today and can be a source of deep and lasting joy, not just in moments of unexpected pain but throughout every minute of your day.

Lord Jesus, I know moments of pain will come. Yet You know the condition of my heart—that I want to choose what pleases You. Thank You for the legacy and everlasting name that You promise me, whether I have children or not. Thank You that it meets my deepest longings. And while I spend this short time on earth, I realize this pain won't always go away, and I rejoice in the hope of eternity. Amen.

ALEX PICKERING

You have a legacy and an identity from the Lord, irrespective of what the future brings.

Turning to God
in Everything

———— 12 ————

The wisdom from above is first pure, then
peaceable, gentle, open to reason, full of mercy
and good fruits, impartial and sincere.

JAMES 3:17 ESV

My husband, Chad, and I can't have kids. We *really* tried. Years now after our last negative pregnancy test—our infertility journey with a surrogate ending with the loss of our three embryos, our three babies—I can say that although this journey lives with us forever, it doesn't define us. When people ask me how we got to this point, I tell them we turned toward each other, and we turned toward God. And with every turn toward Him, He met us with His wisdom.

When we turn toward God, this path through infertility doesn't have to define us. We must turn toward Him with our doubts, fears, and the anger we feel at having to go through this. We must turn toward Him with every decision, test, procedure, medicine, and bill. We must turn toward Him *first* every time, take Him at His word, and allow His wisdom to become promises, guidance, and truth to us.

Turning to God in all these moments doesn't mean the

path ahead won't be hard. What it does mean is that we will have an empathetic and loving Companion for the journey, a God we can trust because He is the character behind the kind of wisdom James 3 talks about. Our God is pure and the provider of peace. He loves us gently and fiercely, more than we can imagine. Our God is fair, even when life isn't. His heart is full of mercy and grace toward us. He makes the journey fruitful and for our good. He gives us dignity and honor despite our circumstances.

Whatever doubt, fear, or decision we face, God is ready with His wisdom—and this wisdom is first and foremost His good and loving presence with us.

Father God, Papa, sometimes You are the last person I turn to, especially when things are hard and dark. Help me to turn toward You first in full trust. Help me to know that when You seem quiet and it is dark, it often only means You are so very close. Open my eyes and my heart, Lord, to Your wisdom, truth, and most of all, love. Amen.

JUSTINE FROELKER

*What do you need to turn toward God
or each other about today?*

Easy Answers

——————— 13 ———————

My ears had heard of you but now
my eyes have seen you.

JOB 42:1–6

Y ou just need to relax, and then it will happen."

"Have you tried zinc supplements?"

"Everything happens for a reason."

Maybe like us, you've had a few of these cliché suggestions slapped like a Band-Aid on the gaping wound of your infertility. While most who share them mean well, in our experience the answers to our problems are rarely so simple.

The experience of unhelpful advice is nothing new. Some believe the story of Job may be the oldest in the Bible. Among the wreckage of his life, Job had a handful of friends who stayed in silence with him for days (Job 2:13)—much better than the few seconds most people last! Eventually, though, their discomfort moved them to offer easy answers to Job's pain:

"God must be punishing you."

"There must be sin in your life."

"You just need to repent."

When God finally spoke, He condemned their ignorant

talk and, through a head-spinning tour of the cosmos, showed just how limited human understanding is (chapters 38–41).

Instead of easy answers, God gave Job no answer at all. Instead of providing knowledge, God invited Job to know Him personally. This encounter moved Job's faith from secondhand information to firsthand experience: "My ears had heard of you but now my eyes have seen you" (42:5). God also restored to Job the consolation of friends and family (42:10–11) because a neat answer will never give the comfort the presence of others can.

Job's story shows that God gets as annoyed with easy answers as we do. He also knows that what we really need isn't to know the answers but to know Him. In our suffering, He invites us into a deeper relationship. The invitation is there for both of us today.

Father God, like Job I have been offered easy answers and at times have questioned where You are in it all. Lord, like him, may I be able to say through this trial, "My ears had heard of You but now my eyes have seen You."

DAVID LOWRIE

In our suffering God offers His presence, not simplistic answers.

From Problem
to Mystery

———— 14 ————

Surely I spoke of things I did not understand,
things too wonderful for me to know.

JOB 42:1–6

My husband, Tim, is shopping averse—and not because he'd rather not spend money. The crowds, choices, and bright lights can leave him miserable with a headache by the end of the day. Our solution to this has been to relabel our shopping trips as "dates in the city." This has focused the task on our time together, and incorporating a special lunch into the day has provided an added blessing. Relabeling the occasion has reduced the stress involved.

In a similar way, Tim and I were stuck with the stress of infertility until we realized relabeling might help change this experience too. We had labeled our situation "a problem," which raised hard questions like, Why is this happening to us? What have we done to deserve it? Wouldn't we make good parents? So we started talking instead about what relabeling might be needed here.

I began by relabeling myself as a "finite creature" with limited knowledge—rather than "God," whose place I was in danger of taking given my judgment that He'd done so wrong by me. I humbly confessed this mistake, vowing to trust He had my best interests at heart.

The second, and most effective, relabeling came from observing how Job wrestled with hard questions during his own suffering. His wrestling seemed to end when his "problems" became "mysteries" in God's loving hands. Notice how God never answered Job's questions but rather gave Job an accurate view of Himself (Job 38–41; 42:1–6). So I stopped striving to understand things beyond me and started trusting the One for whom my infertility was not a mystery.

The result? Relabeling my problems as mysteries has brought peace and even joy.

All wise and loving Father, would You grant me peace of mind to trust You with these hard and painful things I cannot understand? Show me how You are enough to fill all the holes in my understanding. While Your ways of working are so often mysterious to me, I will rest assured today You are working out something glorious. Amen.

DORCAS BERRY

How could relabeling your problems as mysteries help you leave them in God's hands?

Boundaries

When Jesus heard what had happened, he
withdrew by boat privately to a solitary place.
MATTHEW 14:12–13

My phone pinged with a text:

"I understand. Thank you for letting me know. I really appreciate it."

For weeks I had been tying myself in knots trying to figure out how to get out of my friend's baby shower. I had no illnesses, no prior engagements, no easy reasons I could give. But I knew deep in my heart I couldn't face going. The idea of joining in games and putting on a happy face made me feel physically ill. I knew I was too fragile, so I decided to text my friend and be completely honest—telling her it would be too much for me. The fear of offending her was great, but her response showed that my honesty had helped deepen our friendship.

When Jesus learned about the death of John the Baptist, he sought solitude, taking Himself away to grieve and process (Matthew 14:12–13). There will probably be many times when you need to withdraw or seek solitude, too, as you navigate infertility. There may be baby showers, baptisms, birthday parties, men's or women's groups (that are more like dads' or moms' groups) that you don't feel strong enough to attend. That's okay. While it's important not to pull away from all community, learning to recognize what you need and have capacity for is important.

Navigating relationships can be tricky at the best of times, let alone when you're going through this. Giving yourself permission to say no to specific events or to make space for the grief you're experiencing is a good starting point.

Which situations do you find most difficult to face? Where are you longing for some space for yourself? Honestly stating what you need may seem daunting, but it may surprise you how it will help you build connections.

Dear God, I want to show up and be present, but some situations are difficult to deal with. Give me wisdom about where I should spend my time. Help me to find the words to express what I need. Fill me with Your strength and peace. Amen.

SHEILA MATTHEWS

_____

Is there an upcoming event you're dreading to attend? How could you open an honest conversation about it?

Emoji Hearts

—————— 16 ——————

*That is why a man leaves his father and mother and
is united to his wife, and they become one flesh. Adam
and his wife were both naked, and they felt no shame.*

GENESIS 2:24–25

O ut of nowhere my wife exploded, "I hate the hearts!"
Trying to be helpful and fun, I had placed red emoji hearts
on our calendar to mark peak fertility days, when it was "go
time" for us intimacy-wise. Unfortunately, those hearts made
Kelley feel pressured, frustrated, even angry.

I never could have prepared for how much our intimacy
would be impacted during infertility. We became so focused
on the act and the goal that we forgot about the heart, the
love, and the point of intimacy. Sex became merely a means
to an end—to create the baby we longed for.

Genesis 2:24–25 describes husbands and wives becoming
"one flesh"—intertwined in mind, soul, and body—through
sexual intimacy. In God's design, sex isn't supposed to be a
duty or a task to check off but how we as couples express
our oneness. Like Christ and His church, we are united
(Ephesians 5:31–32).

How can we maintain this purpose for sexual intimacy
when infertility often turns it into a task? We can start by

openly discussing our feelings and what we need from each other. We can initiate sex at unexpected times, just for the sake of being together. Some couples even take breaks from trying to conceive, to help them focus on each other rather than pregnancy. We'll need to have grace for each other, as we won't always get it right, but infertility doesn't have to rob us of connection and love.

As helpful as marking peak fertility days can be, "emoji heart" moments can soon become linked with pressure, frustration, and disappointment when failure to conceive follows. Beyond planned sex with pregnancy in mind, let's approach our spouses without expectation, making intimacy romantic and fun again.

Father, this season has been hard in so many ways, including this area of intimacy. As we draw closer to You during this time, may we also be drawn closer to each other. Renew our desire for each other physically as we seek to stay united. I pray that our marriage and intimacy becomes stronger as a result of our infertility journey.

JUSTIN RAMSEY

How can you keep oneness as the goal of sexual intimacy, not just conception?

Grief and Joy

"Don't for a minute think I'm a bad woman.
It's because I'm so desperately unhappy and
in such pain that I've stayed here so long."

1 SAMUEL 1:9–16 MSG

It took six years of infertility and four miscarriages before I realized I was grieving. I had somehow come to believe I couldn't grieve a baby I'd never met or held. But you only have to read the guttural pain in Hannah's prayer to know that the grief of infertility is not only very real but also entirely legitimate and extremely complex. Hannah was "crushed in soul," cried "inconsolably," and was "desperately unhappy" as she poured out her heart to God (1 Samuel 1:9–11, 15–16 MSG).

The grief of infertility is complicated because it doesn't resolve neatly, which is why it's so tiring. It's a hidden grief, which is why you feel so lonely. And it's a disenfranchised grief, which is why you may feel guilty or frustrated, because this world rarely acknowledges the pain of infertility. But Hannah's prayer was included in the Scriptures to show that you are not alone, it's okay to grieve, and your own story of it matters.

Grief cannot be contained—trust me, I've tried. It has to be expressed. Everyone grieves differently, whether they write it out or weep it out, express it in the presence of a friend, in the back row of a church, or just alone. Grieving is the decision to make space for your soul to declare in the presence of God, "This is unfair. This hurts, but I place my pain in the hands of the God who defeated death. I declare in faith that my suffering will not have the final say."

God promises joy to the grieving (Psalm 30:11), but to receive it we must first acknowledge our pain. If you haven't had a good cry recently, perhaps it's time for one.

"How long, Lord? . . . How long must I wrestle with my thoughts and day after day have sorrow in my heart?" (Psalm 13:1–2). "I remain confident of this: I will see the goodness of the Lord in the land of the living" (Psalm 27:13). With You, God, I can face the darkness of the valley as I search for hope once more. Amen.

LIZZIE LOWRIE

Expressing your grief to God and others makes room in your soul for fresh trust.

The Human Part
of Miracles

———— 18 ————

"How many loaves do you have?"
he asked. "Go and see."
MARK 6:35–44

When my friend and her husband struggled to conceive, doctors recommended she have her fallopian tubes flushed. But she was hesitant. "Shouldn't we just pray," she said, "and if I don't get pregnant, see that as God's will?" My friend was trying to figure out how human action and God's intervention work together. I resonated with her query, having wrestled myself with knowing God's will in whether Merryn and I should try IVF or wait for a miracle.

I found help in the story of Jesus miraculously feeding thousands of people with just a little bread and some fish (Mark 6:41–42). Notice who fed the crowd. It wasn't Jesus but the disciples (v. 37). And who provided the food? The disciples did (v. 38). Who distributed the meal and cleaned up afterward? Again, it was the disciples (vv. 39–43). Jesus did the miracle, but He did it through the disciples' actions, blessing what they had in their hands.

This divine-human partnership is God's general way of

working. While the crop comes from God (Psalm 65:9–10), the farmer must work the land. While God won Israel's wars (Joshua 10:42), Israel still had to fight them. Human action was required for some biblical miracles, too, such as Peter casting his net for the miraculous catch (Luke 5:4–6) and the blind man washing his face to see (John 9:1–7). God could harvest a field, win battles, open our eyes, or feed crowds without our involvement, but instead He chooses to incorporate our actions into His work.

My friend went through with the fallopian tube procedure and got pregnant a few months later. God's miracles often come by praying and using the ethical options He's placed in our hands.

Lord, thank You for including us in Your work in the world and inviting us to participate in Your miraculous acts. Show us which options are right for us to try; bless what You've placed in our hands and turn it into provision. Amen.

SHERIDAN VOYSEY

God works as we pray and act.

Peaceful Surrender

19

In her deep anguish Hannah prayed to the LORD.
1 SAMUEL 1:9–20

The story of Hannah praying desperately for a child is one many couples trying to conceive turn to for comfort. It's a story that has guided me greatly.

We're told that, after her anguished prayer, Hannah conceived and had a son, Samuel, whom she dedicated to the Lord (1 Samuel 1:11, 20). In this case Hannah's childlessness was God's setup for a miracle. Through her, God brought a key character into the biblical story—Samuel was the first of many prophets who would anoint kings and shape the future of Israel and the world. In this sense, Hannah's story is unique and not something we should expect God to repeat for us. But I wondered, was there something in her actions I could follow?

I would have given *anything* in this world to be a mother. But just as Hannah gave her dreamed-of baby to the Lord, I felt the need to sacrifice my heart's desire for a child and offer it back to Him too. This was a painful act because I knew it meant possibly giving up what I desperately wanted. Was I prepared for that? After struggling for a long time, I

37

eventually surrendered this dream to God. I then did what I knew God had called me to do, which I'd so far resisted—enroll in theological college. A short while later, I discovered I was pregnant.

There are no formulas in the Christian life for getting what we want. Some couples will surrender their dream of a child to God and not get pregnant. The decision is His.

The peace I found once I'd submitted my will to God was overwhelming. I was ready to follow God wherever He took me, knowing it was the best place to be. Peaceful surrender to His will was another blessing He birthed within me.

Lord, help me to surrender my heart's desires to You, knowing I can trust You with them. May the roller-coaster ride of emotions that infertility brings be translated into new levels of worship to You. In Jesus' name I pray, amen.

ANGELINE LEONG

Invite the Holy Spirit to help you peacefully surrender to God's will for you.

Breaking Traditions

——————— 20 ———————

"The two will become one flesh."
EPHESIANS 5:21–31

A wedding is supposed to be the most magical moment of a person's life. Well, mine was. I married my beautiful wife, Daisy, at the church she grew up in. Looking back now, I see that day as not only magical but as the day we also broke away from Filipino tradition.

A Filipino wedding is often lavish, with dancing and a bountiful spread of delicious food. But Daisy and I decided to keep things practical, having a small wedding with just a few friends and family. The magic of our wedding day would come from its love and honesty, not from traditional pomp and festivity.

A couple of years later, Daisy and I would again break tradition by failing to satisfy people's expectations that we would have children by then. Modern, high-tech Philippines still has a pull toward the traditional, and a Filipino family is typically defined as a father, mother, *kuya* (older brother), *a-te* (older sister), and baby. If your family doesn't fit this formula, you're considered incomplete or even cursed. These notions can lead to embarrassment for a couple struggling to conceive, and the pressure to conform is enormous. Even though we've now built our family through adoption, people still ask us why we remain "childless."

What is marriage? It is the union of two souls before God, each member bound to the other through mutual love and sacrifice (Genesis 2:18–24; Ephesians 5:21–31). This is good to remember when the pressure to conform comes. Faithfulness to God and each other is the essence of marriage, not the fulfillment of family or cultural traditions.

Daisy and I have gotten used to being labeled the "non-traditional couple"—and we love it! May you, too, be free to enjoy your marriage, even when it fails to meet others' expectations.

Dear Lord, thank You for the gift of marriage. Help us to always see what it is about—the union of two souls in Your name. With Your love, help me to cherish my life partner, even if it means going against traditional expectations. Amen.

EDWIN ESTIOKO

Marriage is the two of you—plus God!—against the world.

Brokenness and Beauty

— 21 —

Religion that God our Father accepts
as pure and faultless is this: to look after
orphans and widows in their distress.

JAMES 1:27

My story begins overseas, where I was adopted as an infant. Later, my own children would join our family through international adoption as well. Experientially, I know multiple layers of the loss involved in adoption—both as an adoptee and as an adoptive mother. I may never know certain aspects of my history or my children's. But those pieces aren't unknown to the Lord. Adoption may be born out of loss, but God promises He'll redeem the brokenness.

Many of our personal stories include difficult and challenging circumstances for which we may have unanswered questions and longings. In the middle of brokenness and loss, God promises to heal the brokenhearted and bind up their wounds (Psalm 147:3). Adoption is much like the Christian faith—walking by faith and not by sight. As we navigate all the joys and sorrows of life, we do so with the Spirit, who helps and intercedes for us in our weakness (Romans 8:26).

Christians are beneficiaries of the greatest adoption in history (Romans 8:15). Because of the finished work of Christ on the cross, we are adopted into God's family as His sons and daughters. Our spiritual reality reshapes our earthly experiences and tells us a truer and better story about ourselves and our future.

James 1:27 calls us all to care for orphans. While that doesn't mean all are called to adopt, some are called into the brokenness and beauty that is adoption. If that is you, may we both walk the path of adoptive parenthood with our gaze on the God who promises to never leave or forsake us.

Father, throughout Scripture we learn of Your care and concern for the fatherless. I know that each person is "fearfully and wonderfully" made in Your image (Psalm 139:14), and I need wisdom to discern how You are calling me to care for the vulnerable. Give me wisdom, strength, grace, love, and compassion as I surrender to Your path and plan for my life and how You are creating my family.

CHELSEA SOBOLIK

Adoption is one of God's powerful ways of bringing beauty out of ashes.

The Strength of Weakness

22

"My grace is sufficient for you, for my power is made perfect in weakness."

2 Corinthians 12:6–10

My wife, Julie, squeezed my hand so tightly I thought it might break. I stood by her hospital bed as the doctor took a sample of her uterine wall for further testing, and I could see the pain on her face and feel her discomfort as I held her hand in mine.

How many more things like this do we have to go through? I silently moaned, smiling at Julie and trying to reassure her that everything was all right. It wasn't. At least not for me. I may not have been the one undergoing these invasive procedures, but my heart was breaking for my wife. Was it supposed to be this difficult? I wanted to do something to ease her pain, to fix all this, to protect her.

It's hard to be the strong one in those moments when you're sharply reminded of your helplessness and inability to mend situations beyond your control. Sometimes I just want it to go away. Yet I am reminded of Paul, who pleaded with the Lord to remove the thorn in his flesh—and the unexpected reply from Jesus: "My grace is all you need. My power works best in weakness" (2 Corinthians 12:9 NLT). Amazingly, it is in my weakness that I am *better* equipped to comfort my wife, extending to her the grace that's given to me.

Infertility has a way of amplifying our shortcomings, and I often wonder if I'll be ready to stand up to the challenges. But I can stand firm on God, my rock and fortress (Psalm 31:2), who gives me confidence to face any difficulties that come our way. Whenever I'm feeling empty and weak, I tell myself it's okay because in those moments, I actually have everything I need. I can be strong for her because He is strong for me.

Lord Jesus, I turn to You as my protector and my safe fortress. Guard my heart against feelings of inadequacy and strengthen me to be a safe refuge for my spouse when they need protecting the most. Teach me to embrace my weakness because Your grace is all I need. Amen.

NICHOLAS RICHARDSON

Like water filling a jar, welcome the Lord's strength into your weakness today.

A Firm Foundation

23

*I pray that you, being rooted and established
in love, may have power, together with all the
Lord's holy people, to grasp how wide and long
and high and deep is the love of Christ, and to
know this love that surpasses knowledge.*

EPHESIANS 3:14–19

My husband, Jon, and I are in the process of converting an old barn into a home. When the builders first started, it took them several weeks to take the building apart. To any bystander, it would've looked like a demolition, not a renovation.

There was one wall that, once construction started, we realized would have to be demolished and rebuilt because it had no foundation. The rebuilding process began with making sure the foundation was laid correctly. From this strong base a new and beautiful wall has been built back.

Much like the wall of our barn, our journey through infertility caused me to deconstruct my faith. I found myself questioning who God was and how He acts in my life. Our struggles took me right back to the foundation of my faith.

And what is that foundation? It's God's love for us. In his prayer for the Ephesian church, the apostle Paul prayed that they would *know* this love (Ephesians 3:14–19). We tend to think of knowledge in a cerebral way, but in the Bible, to "know" something is relational and experiential, like how we "know" our loved ones. When we are struggling with all the questions and doubts infertility brings, we need to experience God's love, to root ourselves in it. It's the foundation upon which our faith is built.

When we start from the foundation of knowing we are loved, rather than demolishing our faith, times of pain can lead to faith renovations, where we emerge with a faith that is deeper rooted and more beautiful than it was before.

Heavenly Father, thank You that doubt isn't the opposite of faith. Help me to experience Your love for me today—a love that is so high and wide and deep I'll never reach its end. Amen.

KATHERINE GANTLETT

———————————————

How will you remind yourself of God's deep love for you today?

Good Things, Right Things

24

*Do not conform to the pattern of this world, but be
transformed by the renewing of your mind. Then
you will be able to test and approve what God's
will is—his good, pleasing and perfect will.*

ROMANS 12:1–2

No one wants to be the person who says no to adoption,
right? Particularly if you're a Jesus-loving, Bible-believing
Christian who knows how much God wants homes to be
opened, arms to be widened, and families to grow in worship of the "father to the fatherless" who "sets the lonely in
families" (Psalm 68:5–6). But there we were, Claire and I, sitting at a table for two, discussing our future over a meal and
saying no to adoption. And you know what? It felt right—a
relief. Peaceful.

Claire and I had finally shared out loud what we had
each been feeling inwardly for months. During the previous
year we had daily sought God on the subject, exploring our
options and hearing amazing stories from parents with firsthand adoption experience. We had petitioned God to give us

a heart's desire for adoption, but if anything, honestly, our desires had gone the other way.

Some ten years on, it still remains hard to admit adoption is a good thing to do but not a good thing for *us* to do. Yet our ongoing peace is a testament to that. Perhaps you recognize similar feelings of awkwardness when facing choices you fear may be hard to justify to others.

There are many good things in this world, but we must discern what is good for us and when. How? By having our minds renewed in God and living in His good, pleasing, and perfect will (Romans 12:2). When we experience His peace through our prayerful decision-making, we can be assured He is blessing our choices.

Father God, Your will for our lives is good, pleasing, and perfect. Join us in our decision-making and open our hearts to the good gifts You have in store for us in this season. Help us to discern when the good things of the earth are not good for us. We trust You. Amen.

CHRIS SANDYS

Not every good thing is right for every person.

No Need to Explain

25

All the days ordained for me were
written in your book
before one of them came to be.

PSALM 139:13–16

I stood in silence waiting for prayer, my hands outstretched, when a member of the church prayer team approached and asked how she could pray for me. I explained that my husband and I, after years of trying to start a family, had recently accepted it would just be the two of us. I told her I was finding it hard to explain to others the invisible grief of infertility and our choice not to pursue IVF or adoption. It felt like others didn't understand or assumed we couldn't have been that desperate for children.

She started to pray, and after a minute spoke these freeing words as if from God Himself to me: *"Others don't need to understand the path I have chosen for you."* I immediately felt the pressure lift. If we were following God's lead, why was I expecting others to embrace our choices anyway? All that mattered was that we were trying to follow God's path for us, to the best of our ability.

Since that moment I have absolved myself of the pressure to explain our childless life to others. If people ask whether we have children, I simply answer, "Sadly, that didn't happen for us." When they want to know more and it's appropriate, I happily tell them. But I don't feel the pressure to make anyone comprehend the whys of our journey anymore. That's between us and God, who has ordained our days (Psalm 139:16).

With so many options around infertility, you, too, may feel the pressure to explain your choices to others when they ask. How liberating it is to know that God asks us only *one* question: *"Do you trust Me?"*

> *God, I want to trust You, but sometimes other voices lead me to question the path You've laid out for me. Help me guard my heart and let through only what is from You. May Your voice and Your Word be the only influences steering my life and our infertility journey. Thank You that Your will for my life is completely unique, tailored just for me. Amen.*
>
> CLAIRE SANDYS

Others don't need to understand God's path for you.

Unchanging

26

*God cannot lie. We who have turned to Him
can have great comfort knowing that He will
do what He has promised. This hope is a safe
anchor for our souls. It will never move.*

HEBREWS 6:18–19 NLV

My breaking point came one day during supper preparations. Seven days late with my period, I was likely only carrying hope and not a child—and when that hunch was confirmed right before supper was served, the ache I felt was so expansive I thought my heart and my dreams of motherhood had been flushed out as well. I was done with the never-ending turmoil of trying to conceive. Monthly pain was one thing; grieving each time was too much to bear.

I tried pursuing other dreams for a while—creative passions like writing and handmade greeting cards—yet they didn't offer smoother sailing. It felt like I was either chasing vapors or giant storms were chasing me. That's when it dawned on me—I was placing my hope in things that could shift with the winds. If I wanted to escape the cycle of constantly crushed hopes, I'd need to anchor my hope in something more certain.

A quick Scripture search held the answer. God is that

anchor (Hebrews 6:19). Written over hundreds of lifetimes, the Bible shows us we can be certain of God because He *never* changes. He is our unshakable hope! When circumstances shift like the seas, we can trust that His promises hold true eternally (v. 18).

His plans for me included a fulfilling future, no matter what happened. With this awareness, I found the courage to start trying for a baby again, knowing I'd found a place of peace should the monthly storms return. Being anchored in God, I knew His plans for me were trustworthy.

Lord, the storms of life are overwhelming sometimes. Help me to remember the wind and waves know who You are and are subject to Your authority. When I am being tossed by the waves and fear grips me, Your immovable presence and unchanging promises give me the hope and courage I need to keep going. Amen.

LORI ALCORN

True hope is found not in the good things of this world but in our unchanging God.

Chapter 27

———— 27 ————

March on, my soul; be strong!
JUDGES 5:19–21

In 2012, Phillips, Craig & Dean released their song "Tell Your Heart to Beat Again." It was inspired by a heart surgeon's true story. Having removed a patient's heart to repair it, he returned it into the chest and began gently massaging it back to life. But the heart wouldn't restart. More intense measures followed, but the heart still wouldn't beat. Finally, the surgeon knelt by the unconscious patient and spoke to her: "Miss Johnson," he said, "this is your surgeon. The operation went perfectly. Your heart has been repaired. Now tell your heart to beat again." Her heart began to beat.[1]

The idea that we can tell our hearts to do something is strange, but it has spiritual parallels. "Why, my soul, are you downcast?" the psalmist said to himself. "Put your hope in God" (Psalm 42:5). "Return to your rest, my soul," said another, "for the Lord has been good to you" (116:7). After beating Israel's enemies in war, Deborah revealed that she, too, had spoken to her heart during battle. "March on, my soul; be strong!" she told it (Judges 5:21), because the Lord had promised victory (4:6–7).

Our capable Surgeon has mended our hearts (Psalm 103:3).

53

So when fear, depression, or condemnation come as we walk infertility's path, perhaps we, too, should address our souls and say, *March on! Be strong! Feeble heart, beat again.*

> *Lord, thank You for being with me in every trial and battle. I don't know what victory is going to look like in this fight, but I trust You to bring it one day closer. Because of Your promised presence, I will command my soul to act bravely today. In Jesus' powerful name I pray, amen.*
>
> SHERIDAN VOYSEY

Because of God's promised presence, you can bravely face whatever challenge awaits you today.

A Hope and a Future

28

*"I know the plans I have for you," declares the
LORD, "plans to prosper you and not to harm
you, plans to give you hope and a future."*

JEREMIAH 29:10–14

One day amid my wrangling, bargaining, confused prayers, I felt the Lord whisper something kind and surprising to me: *Sarah, I promised to give you a hope and a future, not a hope and a baby.*

I recognized the echo of Jeremiah 29:11 in those words, but the lens through which I viewed that verse had been distorted by the disappointment of infertility and the disillusionment of my so far "unanswered" prayers.

From my diagnosis of infertility at the age of eighteen to eventually birthing my son at thirty-eight, you'd have heard me say a thousand times, "If only I knew the end to the story, I'd be able to handle the waiting so much better." But in that moment of the Lord's whisper, I thought, *Hang on, maybe Jeremiah 29:11 is the end of the story.* Was this God offering me a chance to glimpse His heart anew, to see the end from the beginning? In my waiting, wondering, and wailing, I was learning that since God isn't a God of second best, He won't give us a second-best future. This truth was life giving and perspective shifting for me.

Through this scripture God boldly and beautifully tells us the future is going to be okay—He *will* give us hope and a future. And this promise isn't dependent on the outcome of our fertility journeys. I needed to hear that as I waited all those years for my son. Maybe you need to hear it today too.

Friend, we needn't fear the future. God is the author and perfector of our lives. Our story might look different from the one we would have written, but it is still good and it is still hopeful.

Lord, I don't always understand Your ways. I'm so often confused, and sometimes I can't see the way ahead. Please assure me today of Your plans for me, of the abundant life You have in store. Open my eyes to these revelations and put to rest any fear I have of the future. Amen.

SARAH LANG

With or without children, God has hope and a future for you.

Who Will Take
Care of Us?

29

*"Therefore I tell you, do not worry about your life, what
you will eat; or about your body, what you will wear."*

LUKE 12:22–26

I am asked the question regularly. In fact, I have asked this question myself, and you probably have, too, since it's a question everyone in our situation asks: *If we never get to have children, who will take care of us when we're old?* This concern for our future takes us to the heart of God's promises.

Most of us are familiar with God's promises throughout Scripture. He promised to protect us: "The angel of the LORD is a guard; he surrounds and defends all who fear him" (Psalm 34:7 NLT). He promised to provide for us: "And this same God who takes care of me will supply all your needs from his glorious riches" (Philippians 4:19 NLT). He promised to give us a future: "'I know the plans I have for you,' declares the LORD, 'plans to . . . give you hope and a future'" (Jeremiah 29:11). Still, we may wonder how God will fulfill these promises to *us*. As a caregiver to my parents, I have wondered what my life will be like at their age, without children to look after me.

Jesus told us not to worry about our lives, what we will eat or wear (Luke 12:22). Just as God cares for the ravens, He will look after us (v. 24). This applies to our future too. God will not drop off partway through our life's journey, abandoning us in our elder years. He will protect us, provide for us, walk with us to the end of our days.

What has helped me to trust God with the future? Praying scriptural promises like these every day and night, without fail. You might find the practice helpful too. Reading His truth daily, keeping His promises visible, reminds us He is there for us *all* the days of our lives.

Dear Lord, Your Word tells us not to worry about everyday matters or our lives. You promise to provide all that we need in all the days ahead. We trust You with Your promises today. Amen.

CIVILLA M. MORGAN

What scriptural promise can you meditate on to help you trust God with your future?

Think About
Your Thinking

30

*Take captive every thought to make
it obedient to Christ.*

2 Corinthians 10:3–5

A recent study has shown that we have around six thoughts every minute. That makes over six thousand thoughts in the sixteen or so hours we're awake each day.[1] Another study suggested that around 80 percent of our thoughts are negative and around 95 percent of them are repetitive.[2] That's a lot of negative thoughts circulating in our brains each waking day.

Our minds can be a battlefield of negativity, and this is no less true for people going through infertility. Thoughts of jealousy, anger, frustration, and more can come with alarming frequency, and if left unchecked, they can cause us to spiral down into hopelessness and depression.

How do we combat negative thoughts when they come? The apostle Paul gave us some great advice. "Do not conform to the pattern of this world," he said, "but be transformed by the renewing of your mind" (Romans 12:2). Then in 2 Corinthians he told us to take "captive" every thought and make it obedient to Jesus (10:5).

There were times during our infertility journey when I'd think, *God doesn't care about me. This is so unfair; I don't deserve this.* But recognizing these thoughts for the lies they were, I tried putting Paul's words into practice and replaced my negative thoughts with God's truth instead.

God doesn't care about me was replaced with *God is a good father to me.*

This is so unfair; I don't deserve this was replaced with *God has a good plan for me.*

When we find ourselves going down a negative-thought pathway in our battle with infertility, let's take those thoughts captive and replace them with truth about God—who He is, what He is like, and the good plans He has for us.

> *Jesus, help us keep our thoughts fixed on You. When lies spring up in our minds, help us recognize them and replace them with the truth about who You are and the good plans You have for us, plans You have ordained since before we were born.*

PETE ROSCOE

What recurring negative thoughts do you need to replace with God's truth?

Childless, Not Godless

31

*Both of them were righteous in the
sight of God, observing all the Lord's
commands and decrees blamelessly.*

LUKE 1:5–15

Although years had wrinkled their skin, the flame of faith flickered flawlessly within them. Beneath their stricken years was unwavering confidence in the coming of the Messiah. Luke explained that Zechariah and Elizabeth were "righteous in the sight of God, observing all the Lord's commands and decrees" (Luke 1:6). But the record also states that Zechariah and Elizabeth were childless (v. 7).

In some African cultural and religious settings like mine, it's often believed that the curse of the Lord rests on those who do not have children, or that God is punishing those couples for their sins. Zechariah and Elizabeth's story confronts this stigma, as they are portrayed as righteous and godly. When people learn that I am a pastor and childless, they often add, "Then you're not praying enough." I imagine this callous comment might have been given to the priest Zechariah, too, by those who had never been in his secret audience chamber with the Almighty.

Zechariah and Elizabeth weren't deprived of a child due

to sin or prayerlessness, and the birth of John the Baptist (vv. 13–14) wasn't a reward for their prayer either. They were chosen to bring a major character into the biblical narrative. Being childless does not mean being godless.

Stories of the righteous are sometimes inked with pain on the parchment of sorrows. God's approval of our faith isn't betokened by the gifts He gives us, as even the righteous can be "hard pressed" (2 Corinthians 4:8). Zechariah and Elizabeth enjoyed God's favor in the midst of their infertility. Whatever the outcome of your journey, know that the pain you experience now isn't due to a frown on God's face.

Father in heaven, thank You for the assurance that my infertility is not a punishment from You. Help me to live as a testimony that Your goodness is seen not only when You are giving me things but also when I have received nothing. Help me to see the tokens of Your grace in the bedlam of disgrace. In life's storms, help me be calm as You speak peace. Amen.

SIKHUMBUZO DUBE

God is not frowning on you.

Chapter 32

——— 32 ———

*Look on me and answer, L*ORD *my God.*
Give light to my eyes, or I will sleep in death.

PSALM 13

After our second miscarriage, my husband, Francisco, and I were heartbroken. What's more, we were told we shouldn't try conceiving again for some time. When we finally could, our quest to find doctors who could provide answers—and every month of waiting that followed—brought pain, tears, and at times, hopelessness.

King David expressed similar feelings in Psalm 13. In just two verses he asked, "How long?" four times, feeling like God had forgotten him, the closeness they once shared seemingly replaced by silence and sorrow (vv. 1–2). Yet David trusted God enough to turn to Him again, begging Him to give him light, life, and victory (vv. 3–4). Then, with renewed hope and anticipation, David turned his prayer to praise. God's goodness and love had been evident in the past, and David was confident God hadn't changed. "I will sing the LORD's praise," he ended his prayer, "for he has been good to me" (v. 6).

When Francisco and I had only tears and no more words, we turned to psalms like this and prayed them out loud together. Praying the psalms this way gave us strength, increased our faith, and even brought joy in our waiting. If you'd like to try something similar, we found these psalms particularly helpful to pray aloud: 3, 5, 13, 20, 23, 28, 42, 43, 61, 63, 86, and 142.

When pain and hopelessness seem overwhelming, and when our own words run out, the psalms can become our prayers. As we cry their Spirit-inspired words aloud, like David, we, too, will grow in confidence and anticipation.

Dear God, how long will You forget us? How long will we wrestle with our pain, our waiting for a baby, and all the unanswered questions? Our Lord and our God, please turn Your face toward us, pay attention to our struggles, bring light in our darkness, and answer us. We trust in You, for You have been good to us.

ESTERA PIROSCA ESCOBAR

When your words run out, let the psalms become your prayers.

Finding Purpose

—— 33 ——

The LORD will fulfill his purpose for me.
PSALM 138:1–8 ESV

It is all too easy to fall into feelings of inadequacy when you can't do what it seems everyone else can. Infertility was crushing for me. There was a void of support groups and therapeutic outlets for men like me to seek help from, and comforting my emotionally distraught wife made the grind almost unbearable. It hit my sense of purpose, too, leaving me feeling aimless.

If I have learned anything through this journey, it's that such moments can force us to discern God's bigger purpose for our lives. Our crisis forced me to analyze my beliefs about what being a man and a husband meant and how my world-shaped beliefs about both were negatively influencing me. It was neither easy nor quick, but through focus, prayer, and journaling, I found myself discovering who God calls me to be—a great husband and leader in my community.

Discovering this purpose shifted my priorities. I began to nurture my relationship with my wife, spending time with and becoming more focused on her. I pursued my purpose by being a servant-leader to those around me, loving them the best I could. I came to the ultimate realization that God calls me to be a source of peace to others, honoring Him by honoring them, bringing encouragement in the face of difficulty. Living this newfound purpose gave me contentment and joy I didn't know I could have.

What is God's bigger purpose for you? Though you may walk in the midst of trouble now (Psalm 138:7), know the Lord wants to fulfill this purpose for you (v. 8). Sharing His steadfast love with others is key to finding the answer.

Father God, help me to know Your purpose for my life—as a spouse, a colleague, a friend, a believer. Grant me calm in the midst of the storm and help me to spread that peace to others, becoming a rock of rest while I remain resting in You. Amen.

THOMAS NEWTON

Your purpose is not defined by your fertility but by the One who loves you.

Body Strength

34

From him the whole body, joined and held together
by every supporting ligament, grows and builds
itself up in love, as each part does its work.

EPHESIANS 4:10–16

Do we have to?" I grumbled. My husband, Colin, gave me a patient *we've-already-been-through-this* look and replied, "Yes. We need it." We had just started attending a new church and were on our way to our first life group get-together. Colin thought we should go to meet other couples. I thought a root canal sounded more fun than a dinner party with strangers who probably all had kids.

Infertility can complicate our relationship with church, causing us to feel disconnected and also making us want to disconnect. We might think we don't belong in such a traditional, family-centric environment. Sunday services expose us to moms patting their baby bumps and fathers shushing their children—sights and sounds our hearts ache to experience. So to avoid the shame, awkwardness, and pain, we opt out.

But as believers church is vital to our well-being. Paul called the church the body of Christ (1 Corinthians 12:27). God designed us to function best when we live interdependently with other Christians. We build each other up (1 Thessalonians 5:11), worship and pray together (Acts 2:42), and bear one another's burdens (Galatians 6:2). Imagine a nose trying to breathe on its own. Neither can we thrive without our fellow Christians.

Colin was right—we needed church community. Despite my reluctance, that life group dinner introduced us to people who became dear friends and faithful supporters through our infertility journey. Though it's hard when we're hurting, we need to stay connected with church. We can find strength beyond our means in the body of Christ.

Lord, You hold me together even as my dreams crumble. I know church is Your idea, yet I sometimes struggle feeling at home there. Help me believe that You designed the body of Christ for my good. Give me courage to pursue connection at church so I can grow closer to You. Thank You for making me part of your Spirit-powered support network.

JENN HESSE

Church community keeps us thriving.

Reframing Mother's Day

35

*He comforts us in all our troubles so
that we can comfort others.*

2 CORINTHIANS 1:3–5 NLT

My husband, Nick, struggles with going to church on Father's Day. I struggle going to church on Mother's Day. It's difficult to attend when these services focus on celebrating and honoring the very people we long to be—parents.

When I have attended church on these days and been met with the inevitable "Happy Mother's Day!" I've smiled and said, "Thank you" but felt the hurt inside. The well-intentioned greeter doesn't realize the depth of pain just below the surface. At the height of our fertility treatments, a counselor suggested we skip attending church on these dates, which was good advice.

During this difficult period the Lord comforted me through my friend Cindy, who began a tradition of bringing me flowers every Mother's Day. Her outward focus moved me because she carried her own grief—the tragic loss of her fiancé in a workplace accident years ago. Cindy's sensitivity was birthed out of her pain, and her thoughtfulness brought profound healing to me.

Now, years later, Nick and I try to imitate Cindy's thoughtfulness. When we attend church on Mother's and Father's Day, we reach out with cards or gifts to those in our congregation who are hurting. One Mother's Day I gave a devotional book to a friend who was struggling in her marriage. She sent me a text later that week explaining how her depression had been replaced with a wave of calm as a result.

Words can't describe the joy that has come from being God's agents of comfort to others (2 Corinthians 1:4). If we hadn't experienced the thoughtfulness of a friend in our time of sorrow, we wouldn't be the people we are today—a couple seeking to lift the spirits of those in need.

Lord Jesus, I thank You for being my comforter. You see me, You hear me, and You know the pain I carry. Please help me to see Your care for me. And even in the midst of my own sorrow, show me how to see the pain of others and pass on the comfort You bring to me.

JULIE RICHARDSON

Whose spirit can you help lift today?

Bless the Way
God Blesses

36

"The LORD bless you and keep you;
the LORD make his face shine on you and be
gracious to you;
the LORD turn his face toward you and give
you peace."

NUMBERS 6:24–26

The longer my wife and I struggled with infertility, the less we spoke about it—or even prayed about it. It was all too painful and so often ended in tears. It became almost as taboo for us to talk about our infertility as others felt talking about it to us! And so we ignored the matter, building a self-protective wall of silence and separation that only served to isolate us from each other. When it came to handling our infertility, we were in different universes.

Then someone suggested we learn to bless each other the way God blesses us. The model for this is found in Numbers 6, where God blessed His people not through giving gifts or acts of service but by simply being present—His face shining on them and turned toward them (vv. 22–26). Knowing God is for you and favoring you, that He's smiling on you and attentive toward you, is a profound blessing, and all the more true now that we've been saved through Christ.

When facing pain and hardship, why do we often turn away from others and in on ourselves? Surely this isolating response is part of living in a broken, sinful world. Instead of turning away from our spouses, we can bless them the same way God blesses us—by turning our face toward them, by smiling, empathizing, being attentive, and letting them know we are there and in it with them, not just as a one-off event but time after time, day after day.

So today let's actively turn our face toward the one God gave us, blessing them with our presence rather than turning away.

Father God, how blessed I am as You turn Your face toward me, assuring me of Your presence and favor, Your attentiveness and care. May I know this great blessing more and more, then pass it on to my spouse—blessing them the way You bless me. May my face shine on them today, Lord, reflecting Your grace and favor. Amen.

TIM BERRY

Bless your spouse today by turning your face toward them, being attentive, responsive, present.

Training for Triumph

37

*Consider it pure joy, my brothers and sisters,
whenever you face trials of many kinds.*

JAMES 1:2–4

I sat there, my eyes welling up with tears and my thoughts lost in despair. Here I was at the hospital again, about to have my third round of surgery. The doctor explained the procedure, but his words offered little hope. I went ahead with the procedure, my longing propelling me to try again.

After the operation, I was wheeled into a ward with two women who had just given birth through C-section. As they chatted about their newborns, I felt the pain of being twelve years married without a child. In my African culture, being a childless woman carries intense stigma. The great African theologian John Mbiti described that stigma this way: "Unhappy is the woman who fails to get children, for whatever other qualities she might possess, her failure to bear children is [considered] worse than committing genocide."[1]

I sometimes feel the chill of being a childless African Christian. When I do, I have learned to remind myself of this: while infertility is a thorn in my flesh, God's power is made perfect in my weakness (2 Corinthians 12:7–9). And while this is a trial I wish I didn't have, James said I can "count it all joy" because, in God's hands, the trial is producing something powerful in me (James 1:2–4 ESV). When I do this, my trials can become teachers that train me to triumph, and my wounds become weapons that withstand the wiles of the wicked one.

Today, may God take your trial of infertility and make it a source of maturity, perseverance, and victory in faith for you too.

> *Dear God, You know how I sometimes feel low. You know how I become angry and confused. Help me count all trials in my life as joy. In facing infertility, may my faith be fortified by Your grace. Amen.*
>
> SONENI DUBE

Consider trials as teachers that are training you to triumph.

My Best Friend

38

*Greater love has no one than this: to lay
down one's life for one's friends.*
JOHN 15:12–13

When I was young I told my grandma I wanted the hymn "There's a Friend for Little Children" sung at my funeral. I loved everything it described—a home of peace and joy, a love that never dies, a crown of brightest glory, a song that never wearies even though it's sung constantly. It was packed with things that thrilled me and a Jesus I longed to be with one day:

> There's a Friend for little children
> Above the bright blue sky,
> A Friend who never changes,
> Whose love will never die.[1]

When Chris and I found out we were facing infertility, a sadness grew in me at the prospect of not being able to pass down the blessings and memories I'd had as a child, like this hymn. Over the years, my faith got complicated, too, by conflicting theologies and confusion around my gifting and calling. Brought back to its words as an adult, I realized my relationship with Jesus had lost the childlike wonder and simplicity expressed in that hymn:

> *Unlike our friends by nature,*
> *Who change with changing years,*
> *This Friend is always worthy*
> *The precious Name He bears.*[2]

Stripping everything back, I've come to cherish again a simple faith grounded in a friendship with Jesus. Jesus chooses us as His friends (John 15:15–16)—what an honor. He said the greatest love was to give your life for a friend (v. 13), which He did for us. Infertility can complicate life and faith, but I'm learning, once again, to rest in the Friend who never changes and on the love that never dies.

Jesus, friend of sinners, friend of little children, friend of mine, thank You for choosing me as Your friend and giving Your life for me. As friendship is a two-way relationship, help me be a good friend to You and those around me. I want to be seen and known in the same way people saw Abraham: "He was called God's friend" (James 2:23). Amen.

CLAIRE SANDYS

What simple truth about life with God
is it time for you to reclaim?

Surplus Love

39

God's love has been poured out into our hearts
through the Holy Spirit, who has been given to us.
ROMANS 5:1–8

Childless for several years, my wife, Daisy, and I felt we had so much love to share. I know it sounds corny, but we felt we had so much care for each other it was almost a crime keeping it to ourselves.

I work as a writer for a Christian child-sponsorship organization in the Philippines, and one of my tasks is to visit impoverished children, find out about their hardships, and tell their stories. It's wonderful to see them registered in the program and helped. I became personally connected to so many families this way, which was partly where I found an avenue to share our surplus love.

Being immersed in the lives of sponsored children made me want to have one of my own. So Daisy and I decided to sponsor a little girl named Claudee, who was from another island in the Philippines. Claudee became our "daughter," bound not by blood but by our commitment to love her unconditionally. In her correspondence she called me "Daddy," which pulls my heartstrings to this day.

Her use of *Daddy* lifts my thoughts to our heavenly Daddy.

Our connection with God isn't based on biology either, but on a love that is unconditional and eternal (Romans 5:8). I am God's child because He registered me into His family by the precious blood of His Son, Jesus Christ (Ephesians 1:5). As a result, God pours His love into our hearts so we can draw others into His family too (Romans 5:5).

Sponsoring Claudee became one of the most beautiful, fruitful decisions Daisy and I have made as a couple, helping us to share our surplus love. God has poured His love into your hearts, too, and has people like Claudee ready for you to share it with.

Dear Father, thank You for loving us despite our transgressions, offering us forgiveness of sins, and adopting us into Your family. Help us, dear Father, to love others as You have loved us—to care for the sick, the weak, the tiny, the children, and those who have no capacity to pay us back. Amen.

EDWIN ESTIOKO

To whom could you direct the surplus love you have as a couple?

Happy for You,
Sad for Me

—————— 40 ——————

*Rejoice with those who rejoice; mourn
with those who mourn.*

Romans 12:9–16

Wait, don't go in there," Sara said, grabbing my arm. "Anna is passing around an ultrasound photo. She's pregnant. I'm so sorry. I didn't want you to be ambushed."

I stayed put in the other room as nervous energy coursed through me. I felt grateful for Sara looking after me that way but also acute pain at what I could've walked into. *Why can't I just be happy for them?* I wondered. *Why does this have to hurt so much?* I worked out how to leave without causing a scene.

The unfortunate truth is that pregnancy announcements cannot be avoided, and for those experiencing infertility, they can trigger feelings of shame, guilt, envy, and deep sadness. I wanted to be happy at Anna's news, but it was hard. Her gain only amplified my lack.

Romans 12 offers us a glimpse of love in action—the kind of love that rejoices with those who rejoice (v. 15) but that is also *sincere* (v. 9). It's not that I couldn't celebrate with Anna but rather that I needed to acknowledge my own sadness too. Pretending to be joyful is very tiring. I have since learned to say, "I am so happy for you but also sad for me."

To help me process others' announcements more positively, I asked friends to email or text me their pregnancy news instead of telling me in person, and I explained that I found ultrasound photos very difficult to see. These measures gave me space to grieve and work through my emotions so I could offer sincere congratulations in time.

What measures would help you to celebrate with your friends who are pregnant? Trusting them with your needs can pave the way for true celebration.

Loving God, You see the fractures in my heart that ache when I find out about my friends' pregnancies. Help me to celebrate with them in an honest way. Guide me in how to communicate my own experiences, and allow my heart to be okay when I hear news that brings up negative feelings. Bless my friendships with an abundance of mutual love. Amen.

SHEILA MATTHEWS

Sincere love allows space for both joy and grief.

Learning to Lament

———————— 4I ————————

How long, Lord? Will you forget me forever?
Psalm 13

Like many women walking through infertility, I was drawn to the story of Hannah as I could see my pain reflected in hers (1 Samuel 1:15). While (thankfully) my situation didn't entail another wife having babies while I couldn't, I lost count of the number of times I had to congratulate friends or family members on their pregnancies. Many times, like Hannah, I prayed desperate prayers. "Lord, if You give us a child, we'll do _____."

One of the practices I found most helpful when it came to articulating how I was feeling was lament. Biblical scholar Matt Lynch defines lament as "the brutally honest and confrontational expression of distress *before God*."[1] I think we have often believed the lie that, if we're honest about how heartbreaking life can be, it means we don't have enough faith. But in Scripture, it's the people with the *most* faith who lament—people like Hannah, King David, and other writers of the Psalms.

All biblical laments contain similar elements, and Psalm 13 is a good model to follow. First, there's a complaint (vv. 1–2), then there's an appeal to God to intervene based on

His character and promises (vv. 3–4), and finally, there's an expression of trust in Him (vv. 5–6). Crucially, we take our complaints about God directly to Him to sort out.

You might like to try writing your own lament. First, express your complaint as fully and honestly as you can. Then, call on God to intervene based on His character and covenant promises. Finally, end by stating your trust in Him. Remember, your lament is addressed to a loving Father who will respond.

Thank You, Father, that I can be totally honest about how tough this journey is. Thank You that You embrace me as I weep. You promise that You are a loving Father who gives His children good gifts. I need to experience the truth of this, to know that You have not forgotten me. Today, I choose to trust in Your unfailing love and Your sovereignty. Amen.

KATHERINE GANTLETT

What would your own prayer of lament say today?

Five Good Things

Give thanks to the LORD, for he is good;
his love endures forever.

PSALM 107:1–9

According to research, those who are intentionally grateful for what they have report better sleep, fewer symptoms of illness, and more happiness. Psychologists even suggest keeping a gratitude journal to improve our well-being, writing down five things we're grateful for each week—whether seemingly mundane, like waking up this morning, or deeply meaningful, like the generosity of friends.[1] Intentional gratitude offers impressive benefits, helping us to stay strong in difficult times.

In this case science is only catching up with Scripture, which has long promoted the practice of gratitude. From the beauties of creation (Psalm 104) to meals and marriage (1 Timothy 4:1–5), Scripture calls us to see such things as gifts and thank the Giver for them. Psalm 107 lists five things Israel could be especially grateful for: their rescue from the desert (vv. 4–9), their release from captivity (vv. 10–16), healing from disease (vv. 18–22), safety at sea (vv. 23–32), and their flourishing in a barren land (vv. 33–42). "Give thanks to the LORD," the psalmist said, for these are all signs of God's "unfailing love."

Gratitude can be a helpful practice for those of us experiencing infertility, which so often keeps us focused on what we lack. Do you have a notepad handy? Why not write down five good things you're grateful for right now? It might be the meal you just enjoyed or your marriage or, like Israel, God's rescue points in your life. Give thanks for the birdsong outside, the smells from your kitchen, the comfort of your chair, the support of loved ones. Each one is a gift and a sign of God's unfailing love for you.

Father, these days I can be so focused on what I lack. But right now I want to be grateful for every good thing You've brought into my life. Each one is precious, whether mundane or meaningful. And most of all, Lord, I'm grateful for You.

SHERIDAN VOYSEY

What five things are you grateful for right now?

Finding Contentment

———— 43 ————

Rejoice always, pray continually, give
thanks in all circumstances; for this is
God's will for you in Christ Jesus.

1 THESSALONIANS 5:16–18

Pray continually," Paul told us. "For everyone who asks receives," Jesus said (Matthew 7:8). But let's be honest, sometimes it can feel like our prayers fall to the ground unheard. I always thought I'd be a mom. It never occurred to me that I wouldn't be. But after fifteen years of prayers, four failed IVF attempts, being turned down for adoption, and three further failed IVF rounds, it seems this particular prayer was not to be.

And yet I am content today. How?

When Jesus said that everyone who asks receives, He isn't suggesting that we treat God like a slot machine but that we can trust Him to give us the right thing (Matthew 7:9–11). And when Paul told us to pray continually, he was talking about more than personal requests. I started growing in contentment when I realized I needed to stop bargaining with God and instead start being still before Him. In my tears and frustration, I sensed His heart was breaking with mine too.

Paul also said to "give thanks in all circumstances"

(1 Thessalonians 5:18). Like that old chorus, "Count your blessings, name them one by one,"[1] doing this helped put things into perspective for me. I have a wonderful husband, and we have a great marriage. I am healthy, have a job I love, and a lay ministry in church that allows me to offer pastoral care to people of all generations—a huge privilege. I am thankful for walks in the countryside, for extended family, for friends, for holidays. While I have my bad days (don't we all), I've reached a point where I'm okay not being a mom.

Giving thanks in all circumstances can be hard at times, but looking for those nuggets of blessing and giving thanks for them has helped me change my mindset and find contentment.

Dear Lord, help me to give thanks whatever my circumstances. Whether I'm having a good day or a bad one, enable me to count my blessings and give thanks for every single one. Amen.

RACHEL QUINLAN

———————

Contentment starts with gratitude for God and His gifts.

Don't Press Pause

44

*"Build houses and settle down; plant
gardens and eat what they produce."*

JEREMIAH 29:1–14

I'm a planner by nature. Much as I might try, I struggle with spontaneity. For me, part of the enjoyment of a holiday or a party is in the expectation and planning.

Our experience of infertility really messed with my need to have a plan. Could I apply for a new job I knew I would love? Or what about the amazing opportunity to buy an old house that would be a project? What would happen if we were in the middle of the building phase and I got pregnant? All of these what-ifs meant it was tempting to put life on hold.

The temptation to simply sit it out and wait was precisely what Jeremiah was addressing when he wrote to the people of Judah in exile in Babylon. Hananiah, a false prophet, had told them they would return home to Judah after two years. No, responded Jeremiah, the Lord said their exile would last seventy years (Jeremiah 29:10).

Jeremiah encouraged the people to "settle down" into exile instead of constantly looking for the end of it. Essentially, they should get on with life—build houses, plant gardens, get married, all the everyday things (v. 5)—even while trusting that God would keep His promise to return them from exile because His plans for them were plans to prosper them and give them hope and a future (v. 11).

Journeying with infertility can feel like being in exile. But the encouragement of this passage is that, rather than constantly looking to the time when exile ends, we can seize the opportunities that life presents now. Don't put your life on hold "just in case."

Heavenly Father, thank You that Your plans for me are good. Help me let go of my need to know when and how this journey will end. Help me choose to say yes to the life I have now with all its opportunities and goodness. Amen.

KATHERINE GANTLETT

Don't let the what-ifs keep you from living life now.

Endings and Beginnings

45

Trust in the LORD with all your heart
and lean not on your own understanding;
in all your ways submit to him,
and he will make your paths straight.

PROVERBS 3:5–6

I don't know" can be a draining and exasperating answer when it comes to the myriad questions a couple faces about childlessness. Should we try IVF? *I don't know.* Would I like to adopt? *I don't know.* Is God even at work in my life? *I don't know.* When will the questions end? *I don't know!* This was me for most of my thirties as my wife, Claire, and I explored every option to rectify our childlessness.

A chance conversation with an experienced soul inspired what we knew we needed to do—to draw a line in the sand and step over it into life as an intentionally childless couple. We took the advice literally, walking to a beach one afternoon with a notepad and a box of tissues in hand. We prayed, cried, listed what we were leaving behind, shared our hopes for the future, and then physically stepped over the line into our new life.

Five years on, we recognize our line-in-the-sand moment was not the end of our grieving but the beginning of it. We had closed a chapter, and that was hard. But God was beginning another—one without so many unanswered questions.

There are still many things we don't understand, but we have learned God wants us to trust Him with the mysteries and keep moving forward anyway. This is the message of Proverbs 3:5–6, that if we daily submit to Him and lay down our need-to-know ways, He will make our paths straight, no matter how uneven the road.

Father God, forgive me for placing my own expectations, desires, and limited understanding before my worship of You. Keep straightening my path as I learn to walk forward, whether through the valley or over the mountain. Thank You that all my beginnings and endings are planned by You and safe in Your hands. Help me to trust You. Amen.

CHRIS SANDYS

Sometimes our endings are God's beginnings.

Other Gifts to Open

46

A gift opens the way and ushers the giver
into the presence of the great.

PROVERBS 18:16

We know children are a gift from the Lord. The Bible tells us so (Psalm 127:3 NLT). We also know that the Lord doesn't give this gift to every person. But when the Lord doesn't give one gift, I've discovered He offers us other gifts to open.

Now well into the second half of my life, long past what might have been my childbearing years, I look with wonder at the gifts God has given me throughout my life. I see they might not have come if He'd given me the blessing of children.

If the Lord had given me children, I know I wouldn't have been able to cultivate the gifts of writing, speaking, and teaching that have touched the lives of many. Yes, I know other women and men who have children can do many other things too. But I also know myself and my limits. I would not have been one of those people.

If the Lord had given me children, I would not have formed the kind of friendships I have with others whom God has called and equipped for lives like mine—lives that don't fit the usual mold.

With children of my own, I'd likely not have become a

teacher of other people's children. I'd likely not have become a professor and mentor to young people whose lives I've been able to pour into, young people I've watched grow and mature in faith, get married, and raise their own children in the Lord.

These lives, these friendships, and these beloved students—these are the "great" ones into whose presence I've been ushered (Proverbs 18:16) through the gifts God has given me to give to them.

Dear God, giver of good gifts, I ask You to open the womb of my heart in order to receive, nurture, and give life to the gifts You have for me. Usher me into the presence of the great with the gifts that only You can give. Amen.

KAREN SWALLOW PRIOR

When God doesn't give us one gift, He offers others for us to open.

Expecting the Best

47

*We know that in all things God works for
the good of those who love him, who have
been called according to his purpose.*

ROMANS 8:28

You don't have a problem if you have triplets, right?" the doctor said. Having tried to get pregnant naturally for a year, we had decided to seek medical help by increasing my ovulation rate with medication. Not only had that medication worked, but the doctor now confirmed I was pregnant! The question was how many babies I was carrying. Our hearts were full of hope and joy. But our joy didn't last long. My next pregnancy test came back negative.

Our disappointment was immense, and we never wanted to suffer like that again. So we lowered our expectations. While we kept trying for a baby, we started expecting the worst, thinking that if it didn't work out, the pain wouldn't be so great. This was a defense mechanism to protect ourselves, but at some point we realized it was getting in the way of our faith.

The message of Romans 8:28 became a lifeline for us: God is good and He always works for our good. Since God is capable of doing amazing things and since He has plans not to harm us but to give us hope and a future (Jeremiah 29:11), why were we expecting the worst for our lives? We decided to start expecting the best from God instead, whatever His best for us might be.

The fear of being disappointed can rob us of the power and joy of believing in a God who can do all things. Disappointments may still come, but God is still good and will always take care of our hearts.

Lord, thank You for Your kindness and presence, and that You are always watching over me. May my heart rejoice in expectation, knowing that You are good and always work for my good, whatever happens. Amen.

GIULIANNA CORRÊA

Have you lowered your expectations of God to protect yourself from disappointment? What might God whisper to you today in response?

Fruitfulness in Christ

——————— 48 ———————

So that you may live a life worthy of the Lord and please
him in every way: bearing fruit in every good work.

COLOSSIANS 1:9–12

Addison walked into our lives as a lost eleven-year-old boy—from a dysfunctional family where he was ignored at best and neglected at worst. He is now a young adult, and it is through Addison that I've come to learn what being "fruitful" really means.

While being fruitful can include bearing biological children (Genesis 1:28), that isn't its only meaning. The apostle Paul also talked about us "bearing fruit in every good work" (Colossians 1:10). For my husband, Louis, and I, this kind of fruitfulness has come by becoming spiritual parents to others.

Addison is one of many godchildren Louis and I have parented over our two decades of marriage. We have journeyed with him through his darkest moments, like when he was hospitalized for a couple of years due to mental illness. We have brought him back from suicide attempts and loved him into the young adult he is today. Addison recently went back to school and has won many outstanding awards for excellence in his studies. It has been so rewarding to see how far he has come, maturing into a fine young man in Christ, a broken life transformed by God's love.

God's heart for us is that we be spiritually fruitful, something we can *all* achieve with Him. What could that look like for you? It might include parenting spiritual children like Louis and I have or serving people in your church or serving those outside it with the love of Christ. Being fruitful lies in impacting lives and seeing them transformed to the glory of God. As Louis and I discovered, it can be fulfilling and thrilling work to do.

Lord, help me to experience what it means to be fruitful in every way through the love of Christ. Show me how I can reach out practically to the people You place in my path. In Jesus' name, amen.

ANGELINE LEONG

With God, there is no unfruitful life.

Feel It, Express It

Those who sow with tears
will reap with songs of joy.

PSALM 126:4–6

When our struggle to have children started grinding us down, I dug in and found the inner strength I thought my wife needed. I took care of the practicalities and stayed calm and cool when she was overwhelmed. On one particularly dark day, I broke into tears but managed to wipe them away before she saw. And so it remained until the day my coldness broke her. "Why don't you care?!" she yelled. "Why don't you show any emotion? Why is it always only me crying?!"

The suppression of emotion I saw as strength was in fact torturing the very person I was trying to help and opening a rift in our marriage. This stiff-upper-lip mentality had been shaped in me by a dopamine-addicted culture that has a thousand ways to stop feeling anything uncomfortable, and the fact that all my role models had been strong, silent men. If only I had looked to a different kind of hero—to David, the warrior-king-poet, who was as comfortable singing tear-soaked prayers to God as he was protecting a nation.

David's psalms fearlessly express the kind of emotions we spend billions of dollars trying to suppress: "All night long I flood my bed with weeping" (6:6); "My guilt has over-whelmed me" (38:4); "How long, LORD? Will you forget me forever?" (13:1). And whereas our emotional suppression leaves us numb and disconnected, all these psalms end on a note of joyful hope. Joy, it seems, belongs to those who grieve (126:5).

Our Father God is inviting us to feel our feelings and express our emotions to Him because grief is not an illness but a journey—one that ends in the arms of our Beloved.

Father God, sometimes the pain is too much to feel and too scary to express. But I am tired of running and I am ready to feel it all—the ache, the questions, the uncertainty. As I let it all out, would You collect my tears and turn them into a harvest of joy?

DAVID LOWRIE

What has been left unspoken between you, God, and each other?

Outsiders

———— 50 ————

"Do not fear, for I am with you;
do not be dismayed, for I am your God.
I will strengthen you and help you;
I will uphold you with my righteous right hand."

Isaiah 41:8–10

Some years ago I invited a group of women over for dinner but failed to register in advance that they were all mothers. As I served drinks, fairy lights twinkling in the background and floral napkins perched neatly on the table, the conversation landed on the topic of birth stories. Noise in the room escalated as the women animatedly shared their experiences, punctuated with bursts of raucous laughter.

I tried my best to engage in the chatter, acting as if it was the most natural thing in the world to talk about epidurals and C-sections, while internally feeling like an outsider in my own home. Later that night when the women left, my tears flowed.

There were times when Jesus felt like an outsider, His own people failing to receive Him (John 1:11). He found solace by getting away to quiet wilderness places to be with His Father (Luke 5:16), who always received Him (John 11:42).

Jesus' approach is a great reminder that our heavenly Father is always there for us "outsiders."

When my guests went home, I shared frankly with God how the night had made me feel. As I did, a lightness entered my spirit and strength arose in me. Our God is with us, ready to help any time of the day or night (Isaiah 41:10). I have discovered that running to Him may not immediately change the situation, but it can bring strength and deep peace in the midst of it.

> *Lord, I thank You that You long to walk with me through the highs and lows of life, to be my trusted companion and cheerleader. I thank You for the friends who welcome me into their lives even though we might not have the same life experiences. Help me to always run to You as the first port of call in times of challenge.*
>
> MARIA RODRIGUES

God always has space for us outsiders.

A Seat at the Table

──────── 51 ────────

*"On that day you will realize that I am in my
Father, and you are in me, and I am in you."*

JOHN 14:15–21

One of the most challenging aspects of our journey with
infertility was the sense of social isolation. It seemed all our
friends and family were having babies, and conversations
often revolved around pregnancy or young children, leaving
us feeling like outsiders.

As creatures made in the image of a triune God (Genesis
1:26–27), being in community and feeling a sense of belonging is a vital part of what it means to be human. So where do
we find this belonging?

I have a print of Andrei Rublev's famous fifteenth-century
icon of the Trinity hanging above my desk. It depicts the
Trinity as Abraham's three visitors in Genesis 18:1–15. Father,
Son, and Holy Spirit are seated around a table, with an open
fourth place at the front. Some art historians think that a mirror was once glued to this place at the table, meaning that
when the observer looked at this painting, they would see
themselves seated with the Trinity.[1] Isn't that a stunning idea?

In John 14, Jesus explained that through His incarnation
we are included in the Trinity. As the fully divine Son of God,

He is the second member of the Trinity and is "in" His Father. And having become fully human, Jesus in a sense joins us to the Trinity, by us being "in" Him (v. 20). What's more, not only is Jesus in the Father, and we in Jesus, but through the Spirit, Jesus dwells in us. "I am in my Father, and you are in me, and I am in you."

The Trinity is the ultimate expression of community. It is a community of love, joy, and delight, and the place where we find our own true belonging. Through Jesus, we all have a seat at God's table.

Heavenly Father, thank You that when I feel excluded, that I don't belong, the truth is I have a community in which I will always belong—the community of love that is Father, Son, and Holy Spirit. Encircle me in Your triune love today. Amen.

KATHERINE GANTLETT

You are embraced by Father, Son, and Holy Spirit today.

Moments of Reprieve

---------- 52 ----------

You have turned my mourning into joyful dancing. . . .
and clothed me with joy.

PSALM 30:8–12 NLT

Standing in the kitchen in my Wonder Woman apron (yes, I have my own Wonder Woman apron), I glanced at my reflection in the mirror. I had become accustomed to peering into that mirror, searching for some recognition of the former me—the me I used to be before infertility sapped the joy I'd always had.

Home alone and baking, I put some music on. And that's when it happened—a moment of joy rising within, a sense of fun popping its head above the trench of infertility. Suddenly I was twirling, whirling, and singing at the top of my lungs, "I'm having such a good time / I'm having a ball / Don't stop me now!"[1] It was exhilarating, refreshing, wonderful.

I would love to tell you I was singing along to some deeply spiritual song, but, alas, it was a song by Queen. But music is a gift, whoever the artist singing it is, and in that moment the joy I felt was holy. In those three minutes and thirty-three seconds, God turned my mourning into dancing and lifted my sorrow (Psalm 30:11), giving me a garment of praise for the spirit of heaviness (Isaiah 61:3). I found myself worshiping, thanking Him, praising Him for this joy and gladness, and for this moment of reprieve.

If you find yourself stumbling upon such a moment of joy, take it. My goodness, *take it*! Many days we won't find our feet dancing, but it's okay to dive right in to such joy when it presents itself. Ask the Lord for some moments of reprieve as you face infertility, too, however He chooses to bring them. And when they come, go right ahead and twirl, whirl, and sing at the top of your lungs.

Lord, please give me a garment of praise for the spirit of heaviness. I ask for some light reprieve along this journey. With Your help, I long to feel joy despite my sorrow. Please refresh me and give me a private-dance-party moment or two with You soon. Thank You that You're here with me. Amen.

SARAH LANG

There are shortcuts to happiness, and dancing is one of them.
VICKI BAUM

The Essence of Manhood

53

*Become mature, attaining to the whole
measure of the fullness of Christ.*
EPHESIANS 4:11–16

Moving from son to husband and father is the essence of manhood. Man up." Though probably well-meaning, these words from someone on social media left me disturbed. Knowing many godly, responsible men who were single or childless by circumstance, I winced at the idea they were somehow less than men. And being childless myself, I began wondering what the real "essence" of manhood might be.

The idea that one isn't fully a man until he has married and fathered a child is common in many cultures and even in some churches. But how biblical is it? While marriage and parenthood are wonderful callings (Genesis 1:28), they aren't the only callings God gives. Paul encouraged singleness for the sake of the gospel (1 Corinthians 7:32–35) and was probably childless himself. Was he any less of a man?

Interestingly, the Bible says less about manhood than it does about *maturity*. Paul described maturity as being humble, gentle, patient, peacemaking, steadfast in belief, and able to speak the truth in love (Ephesians 4:2–4, 15). At the core of being mature, he said, is "attaining to the whole measure of the fullness of Christ" (4:13). And Christ was both single and childless.

This is good news for our sons, brothers, fathers, and friends, whether single or married, not to mention childless husbands like me. The essence of manhood—and indeed of womanhood—isn't fitting a stereotype but becoming like Jesus. And that's something *all* of us can grow in.

Lord, this journey has me facing all kinds of fears and questioning all kinds of beliefs. Thank You that in Your eyes my essence isn't based on meeting a stereotype, and my value isn't based on having children but in being Yours and growing into Christlikeness. Holy Spirit, would You make me more like gentle, bold, sacrificial Jesus today? Amen.

SHERIDAN VOYSEY

———————————————

Jesus is the essence of manhood and womanhood.

Motherhood Myths

54

God chose the foolish things of the world to
shame the wise; God chose the weak things
of the world to shame the strong.

1 CORINTHIANS 1:26–29

In my Zimbabwean language, isiNdebele, it's common to follow a greeting by asking about the well-being of one's children. After "How are you?" comes "And how are your children?" because it's assumed that every married woman has children to inquire about. Consequently, in many African cultures, motherhood is equated with womanhood. A woman epitomizes her being by attaining the envied status of biological parenthood.

It is hard to live in a society that believes in the "motherhood is womanhood" myth and views childless women like me as second class. The only force able to confront this myth is the gospel, which liberates us from sociocultural stigma and makes us whole in Christ.

If God cares for the little sparrow that flies and the flowers that fade (Matthew 6:26, 28–29), I know He values me more. We need to constantly remind ourselves that we were fashioned in heaven in the image of God (Genesis 1:26–27). Peninnah provoked the childless Hannah so much that she wept so bitterly she couldn't even eat (1 Samuel 1:6–7). When the world torments us like Peninnah, let's refuse to be devalued, for we are fearfully and wonderfully made (Psalm 139:14). Let us walk tall, breaking cultural biases by looking positively at our inadequacies—God chooses the weak things of the world to do His work (1 Corinthians 1:27).

My husband once told me, "Your success is not measured by the babies you could birth but the burdens that couldn't deplete your worth." In the eyes of society, I may be less because I am childless. But in God's sight, I am precious and my childlessness does not equal worthlessness. And what's true of me is true of you too.

Dear God, sometimes I feel incomplete. I sometimes forget the value You have ascribed to me as the voices of society drown out Your gentle, soothing assurance that I am Yours and You are with me. Help me never to fret. May those around me experience the power of Your grace through my life. Amen.

SONENI DUBE

What myth is God's Spirit calling you to renounce today? What stigma is He removing from you?

The Bummer Rule

55

*Don't talk so much. You keep putting your foot
in your mouth. Be sensible and turn off the flow!*
PROVERBS 10:19 TLB

One of the greatest marriage tips my wife and I ever learned was from an infertility conference we attended. The tip is called the "bummer rule." Essentially, this is the art of listening to your spouse when they're expressing hurt, frustration, fear, sadness, or anger about something, and instead of offering a solution or taking offense, simply replying "Oh. Bummer." While the exact words you use aren't so important, what is important is the sentiment they convey, which is: *I hear you and I'm with you in whatever you're going through.*

I often rush to try to fix what's broken, right the wrongs, and solve the problems Julie shares with me. But somehow this usually makes things worse! Instead, I'm learning to listen, to let her know I understand the pain and to encourage her that everything will be all right. *I'm sorry. That's hard. Bummer.*

When Job's friends heard about his distress, their first response was to sympathize and comfort him, sitting with him in silent solidarity for seven days and nights (Job 2:11, 13). But after listening to Job's complaints, they couldn't resist voicing their thoughts on the matter, which in the end God wasn't happy with (42:7). Job was best consoled without words. Most of the time, that's the best consolation we can offer too. Talk too much and we can put our foot in our mouths (Proverbs 10:19 TLB).

If we're too quick to offer our own advice, we may short-circuit what the Lord wants to say to both our hearts. Let's leave room for God to bring *His* healing and wisdom to our fears and confusion by just sitting in the moment together. By applying the bummer rule, we can say so much without saying a word.

Lord Jesus, help me to be quick to listen and slow to speak, leaving room for You to work instead of offering advice where none is needed or desired. Teach me through these times that it's okay not to have all the answers, because You do instead. Amen.

NICHOLAS RICHARDSON

Sometimes listening is the best form of care you can offer each other.

The God I Needed

56

*We had hoped that he would be the one
to set Israel free! But it has already been
three days since all this happened.*

LUKE 24:13–32 CEV

Infertility changed my faith. Like the disciples on the road to Emmaus, I used to think I knew how God worked. Just as they had hoped He would immediately set Israel free (Luke 24:21), I had hoped God would instantly answer my prayer for children. But He didn't, and my disappointment in Him created a distance that began to feel insurmountable.

As my disappointment grew, so did my anger. "I don't believe You love me anymore!" I cried out to God one night. For a while I felt nothing in response. Then in the silence, a still small voice spoke to my broken heart: *Look closer!*

As I sat wondering what this meant, my mind slowly filled with memories of the people in my life and the ways they'd loved me during my infertility—from hugs and chocolate to tear-stained prayers. Rather than fixate on my disappointment, I began to expand my search for God on this unfamiliar road. And just like the disciples, I realized Jesus had been with me all along without me seeing it (Luke 24:30–32). He had been loving me through those who had walked beside me all that time.

Looking back, I think I saw God as more of a genie than a Father who wanted a relationship with me. I wanted someone to fix me, but instead I found a God who wouldn't leave me. I wanted answers, but instead I received God's comfort and compassion through others. It took seven miles for the disciples to recognize Jesus' presence alongside them; it took me several months.

Look closer! Who's walking beside you? God does love you and He is there—channeling His love through the presence of others.

Lord, I had hoped You would answer my prayers for a child by now, but I'm still waiting. I can't always see You in the moment, but I trust You are walking beside me. Give me eyes of faith to see You on the journey. Reveal to me a bigger understanding of who You are and where You're at work. Fill me with Your resurrection hope. Amen.

LIZZIE LOWRIE

How has God channeled His love to you through others?

Faith Through the Fire

———— 57 ————

If we are thrown into the blazing furnace, the God
we serve is able to deliver us from it. . . . But even
if he does not . . . we will not serve your gods or
worship the image of gold you have set up.

DANIEL 3:17–18

Trigger warning: baby loss

After years of struggling with infertility, my wife, Emma, and I were so overjoyed when we finally had a positive pregnancy test. Full of faith, we told our family and friends about our long-hoped-for miracle. Then complications arose, and we found ourselves at the hospital having an ultrasound. After minutes that felt like days, the stone-faced sonographer told us our baby had no heartbeat and had died. Our world came crashing down.

As the sonographer stepped out to give us some privacy, Emma and I dared to pray the boldest prayer of our lives—asking God for a healing miracle for our baby. But there was no miracle, the gray images on the ultrasound machine remained the same. Our faith was rocked.

How do we recover when our best prayers aren't answered as we'd like? I found pastor Bill Johnson's words helpful: "I refuse to sacrifice the revelation that God is always good on the altar of human reason because of my need to make sense of my seemingly unanswered prayer."[1]

This is the kind of faith we see in Daniel chapter 3. The three friends Shadrach, Meshach, and Abednego were tied up and facing death for refusing to compromise their beliefs by worshiping an idol. They knew God could save them but were determined that even if He didn't, they would worship Him anyway. This is the kind of faith that can help us get though infertility—a faith that's not based solely on us having a child but on an unshakable faith that God is good all the time, despite the problems in life we may encounter.

Jesus, help our faith in You to be solid and complete, based on Your eternal goodness and not determined by our circumstances. Help us to trust in You daily as the bedrock of our lives.

PETE ROSCOE

Our faith is built on God's goodness, not our circumstances.

Held by Others

58

When Moses' hands grew tired. . . . Aaron and Hur
held his hands up—one on one side, one on the
other—so that his hands remained steady till sunset.

EXODUS 17:8–13

I started well with the whole prayer thing when our infertility journey began in 2002. Full of hope, confidence, and excitement, we gave it all to God knowing our heavenly Father was with us on this road. Sharing what we were going through with others, we knew they were praying too.

As people of faith, prayer is just what we do, isn't it? In good times and bad, in thankfulness and sadness, talking to God is logical and natural. "Pray continually," Paul told the Thessalonians (1 Thessalonians 5:17), which we know is the ideal.

But as treatments repeatedly failed over months and years, my prayers began to sound more like laments—more desperate, more shouty, brutally honest, and raw. Finally, I found it difficult to pray much at all, which felt like a failure in itself—another one.

When I admitted my struggle to pray to my mum, her response was loving and liberating. "Don't beat yourself up about that too," she said. "Even though you have nothing left, remember others are praying for you, carrying you through, holding you before God." Those words brought some peace to my exhausted heart and enabled me to carry on. Like Aaron and Hur holding Moses' hands up when he grew tired (Exodus 17:12), we were being held in a wave of prayer. Even if I was struggling to feel it, God was listening and somehow working in the midst of it all.

When we feel stuck in a cycle of grief and disappointment, and what we long for seems constantly out of reach, it can be hard to keep praying. In the faith community there will be people we can trust with our struggles and disappointments—Aarons and Hurs to hold up our hands, praying for us when we can't.

Lord, this waiting and longing can be so tiring. Sometimes I feel all out of words. Could You surround me with people of prayer, Aarons and Hurs, to hold up my hands right now? I'm just too exhausted to do it myself. Help me to share my needs with them honestly. And thanks for being with me in this. Amen.

HANNAH SCOTT-JOYNT

This journey is an opportunity to be held by the prayers of others.

Bottle of Tears

59

You keep track of all my sorrows.
You have collected all my tears in your bottle.
You have recorded each one in your book.

PSALM 56:8–10 NLT

If tears could be traded as the currency of sorrow, I'd imagine you'd be pretty rich by now. I know I would be. I lost count a long time ago of how many times I've wept over my empty womb, empty arms, empty nest. The reservoir inside never seemed to be depleted. And time after time it felt like those tears were being spilled, lost, wasted. I usually cried alone, feeling invisible to a world that didn't know what to do with someone like me—feeling like no one cared, including God.

Then one day God drew my attention to Psalm 56:8, to me one of the most beautiful word pictures in Scripture. This psalm showed me that God was a tear collector and had been by my side, noticing everything. My tears were so precious to Him that not one had been spilled or wasted but instead collected in a bottle and recorded in His book. He had been *that* close and attentive the whole time.

I once heard heaven likened to a museum of tears.[1] When I get there I expect to see a shelf full of bottles with my name on them—and another full of bottles with yours. I love this personal touch, our God caring that much for each of us.

Some days I do still cry. But when I do, I now offer my tears to God to go straight into His bottle as an everlasting memorial that He cares about me. And on my windowsill now sits one of my most prized possessions—a vintage, purple glass bottle, my memorial, my bottle of tears.

God of heaven, collector of my tears, I praise You for being so close to those who weep in times of sorrow. Prevent me from mistaking Your invisibility for absence or a lack of care. Through the precious picture of bottles of tears, show me again today how much You care for me and how my suffering isn't ignored in Your kingdom. Amen.

DORCAS BERRY

None of your tears have gone unnoticed.

One Noisy, Joyful Home

——— 60 ———

*He chose us in him before the creation of the world to be
holy and blameless in his sight. In love he predestined
us for adoption to sonship through Jesus Christ.*

<small>EPHESIANS 1:4–5</small>

I remember helping my daughter Claudee with her math assignment one afternoon. She was only six years old then. I got really frustrated when she couldn't understand a simple addition problem. I yelled at her, and she cried. I apologized right away and cried along with her. But I couldn't forgive myself for what I did, and I still struggle even today.

That moment makes me reflect on why my wife and I decided to "adopt" Claudee in the first place. We had been childless for several years, until we decided to take in not just Claudee but also her two siblings and their biological mother, who was young enough to be a younger sister to me and my wife. We decided not to legally adopt the children, so they could keep their biological mom's last name, but it is adoption nonetheless. We all live together in one noisy, joyful home.

Adopting a whole family was such a unique decision that people wondered why we did it. Some went so far as to say it wouldn't work. Well, it's been sixteen years so far, and it's working beautifully. And what has kept us bound together is the inspiration that God gives a big nod to the concept of adoption. Jesus paid a great price on the cross just so God the Father could adopt us into His family (Ephesians 1:4–5).

I love my adoptive family to death. Raising children is fun and full of laughter but is certainly no laughing matter. There are many heartaches. But we have discovered that it's possible to form a family bound by love, not blood, and by grace, not genes—just like the family our Father has brought us into.

Father in heaven, it is only because of Your love and grace that we are saved. Thank You for adopting us into Your own family through Jesus, and please show us how to extend that same grace to others today. Amen.

EDWIN ESTIOKO

God's family is bound by love, not blood, and by grace, not genes.

Laura

61

*Ruth replied, "Don't urge me to leave you
or to turn back from you. Where you go I
will go, and where you stay I will stay."*

RUTH 1:3–18

When my mom died of cancer, I felt the weight of our shrinking family, and my longing for a child became even more acute. I wondered if God would ever fill this void in my heart.

Around that time a young woman in my Bible study group asked if I would mentor her. Laura had been praying for a mentor for years and sensed the Lord prompting her to ask me to be that person. Even though we'd just met, she stepped out in faith. That evening turned into coffee chats, walks, and many Bible studies together.

Then something extraordinary happened. Not only did Laura come to work at my organization, she came to work *in my department*. Laura came to us from a completely different field—human resources at a hospital—but now she was on our team as a video editor, and she and I would produce films and travel on productions together all around the world, leading us to bond even more.

We read in the Scriptures how God takes care of His

people. Jesus asked John to care for his mother when he was on the cross (John 19:27), and God prompted Ruth to remain as a daughter after Naomi lost her husband and two sons (Ruth 1:16). Similarly, God cares for us today. I believe Laura is the Lord's spiritual daughter to me. On the first Mother's Day after my mom passed, Laura surprised me with a beautiful dinner, flowers, and a card that read *Happy Mentor's Day*.

Without kids, I sometimes wonder who will take care of Nick and me in the future. But then I see God's perfect provision for me in Laura, and I'm reminded that He is faithful to provide just what we need when we need it, in ways we might not expect.

Lord, thank You that You see me and promise never to leave me. Thank You for taking care of me. Please open my eyes to see the ways You provide for me. When I wonder what my future will hold, help me to know I can trust You with everything. Amen.

JULIE RICHARDSON

Who could you invest time in as a mentor or friend?

From Deserts
to Gardens

62

The LORD will comfort Israel again
and have pity on her ruins.
Her desert will blossom like Eden,
her barren wilderness like the garden of the LORD.
Joy and gladness will be found there.

ISAIAH 51:1–3 NLT

A wildfire burned dangerously close to our fertility clinic—the smoke was visible from our house. We worriedly prayed for the frozen embryos stored there—including our own—and for the many patients who relied on the clinic as the only local place for treatment.

Firefighters eventually extinguished the fire without any damage to the clinic or the neighboring buildings, but the dense woods that had surrounded the area were transformed. The only remains of the once-towering trees were charred, black trunks. I was struck by how the physical landscape now seemed to match the bleak feelings I experienced as I entered the clinic for appointments.

Several years later, I can still see the scars and scorch marks on the parched land. California drought prevents the tree regrowth we'd hoped to see by now. But each spring, when I shift my gaze down from the trees, I see small clusters of purple lupine and orange poppies peppered throughout the dry fields. The contrast of the bright colors blossoming against the brown grass is remarkable.

Now when I drive through this area, I think of Isaiah 51:3. God promised His people Israel that their ruins would not be wasted. They would be fruitful—"Her desert will blossom"— and have reason to rejoice and be glad.

For some people, fruitfulness and rejoicing arrives in the birth or adoption of a long-awaited child. For others, it comes in the form of new dreams and new purposes. Even when it seems like dryness and barrenness surround us, God gives us the gift of joy through unexpected life and beauty.

Lord, Your Word says that You will restore the barren wildernesses in my life. On the hardest days, help me to believe that You can indeed fulfill this promise, and help me to anticipate the forthcoming beauty and joy You have for me. Amen.

LISA NEWTON

God turns barren lands into gardens of gladness. Walk forward in trust.

Naming and
Shaming Shame

63

---

*For the joy set before him he endured the
cross, scorning its shame, and sat down at
the right hand of the throne of God.*

HEBREWS 12:1–3

In the race of life, I often feel like I'm lagging behind, like
I've stumbled and lost touch with the pack. Everyone else is
racing ahead, marrying and having kids, while I've become
an outsider with no place at the school gate or the dads-and-
lads events. In social situations I tend to withdraw, lacking
confidence, walking around with a nagging sense that I'm
odd and there's something wrong with me. As being a parent
is so central to identity in our culture, I guess it's no surprise
that not being one can feel like a stigma and a disgrace. All of
this is me experiencing a sense of shame.

I'm amazed that Jesus experienced this painful emotion of shame too. On the cross He was made to feel like an
outsider and rejected—He was naked and exposed for all to
laugh at and deride; He was considered a disgrace and defiled,
even accursed and abandoned by God (Isaiah 53; Psalm 22;
Hebrews 13:12–13).

How did Jesus deal with the shame? He scorned it (Hebrews 12:2). He literally shamed shame—laughing at it, writing it off as nothing compared to the joy that was coming after His resurrection. This is how we can combat shame too. It feels like a big ask when all this negativity seeks to define and destroy us. But Jesus put things in perspective and showed us what really matters. And because of what He's done for us, there is nothing less than honor, glory, and joy ahead for us too (1 Peter 1:3–9).

So today may you shame shame, too, looking outward and upward to all the value you have in Him now, and all that's in store for you in Christ.

Lord, You named and shamed shame, keeping Your eyes on the joy that was ahead of You. As I walk this painful path, help me to shame shame, too, laughing it off in comparison to the honor, glory, and joy that is mine through You. Amen.

TIM BERRY

Name and shame shame, whenever it comes.

Shame Grows
in Darkness

-------- 64 --------

Rejoice with those who rejoice;
mourn with those who mourn.

ROMANS 12:9–16

We pressed Send and watched as the little "Sent" sign popped up. Words we had never expected to write were winging their way into the inboxes of our friends and family. We looked at each other wordlessly and exhaled. Whatever responses we received, we had taken a step outside of carrying the weight of infertility on our own.

Romans 12:15 is a call to the Christian community to both celebrate with others and to sit with their pain. Joy does not trump grief. We are called to participate in both. But how can others mourn alongside us if we keep our pain hidden? "We have to tell people," I said to Elis. "I can't carry this around anymore." He agreed. We had reached the point where we knew shame had taken root inside us.

Shame is hard to notice at first. It can look like a need for privacy or a need to process first. But our need for privacy and processing had grown into a need to hide the pain from others. It drained us. So we made a list of people who mattered the most in the world to us, whether near or far, and wrote that email explaining the journey we'd been on and where we'd come to. We explained that we didn't know how to talk about it but wanted them to know, and that we needed their love, prayer, and support. As responses flooded in over the following days, we felt a glimmer of light pierce the darkness of our shame. We were bathed in love.

> *Lord, it's hard not to listen to shame. My heart is broken, but I know You see each tear that falls. You hear every whispered prayer. Draw near to me and help me to be brave. Show me who to trust with our story; give me the words to say and people who can hear them. Light of the world, shine into our darkness. Amen.*
>
> SHEILA MATTHEWS

If you haven't already, which trusted family members or friends could you share your journey with?

Not Like That

65

"How much more will your Father in heaven
give . . . to those who ask him!"

LUKE 11:5–13

H aving tried for years to conceive, Richard and Susan were elated when they became pregnant. Susan's health problems, however, posed a risk to the baby, and so Richard lay awake each night praying for them both. One night, Richard sensed he didn't need to pray so hard, that God had promised to take care of things. But a week later Susan miscarried. Richard was devastated. "Did we lose the baby because I didn't pray hard enough?" he asked me.

On first reading, the parable of the friend at midnight might suggest so (Luke 11:5–13). In the story, a man approached his neighbor (sometimes thought to represent God) for help. "Don't bother me," the neighbor replied, "my children and I are in bed." When the neighbor eventually did help, it was only to get the man off his back (v. 8). Read this way, the parable suggests God will give us what we need only if we badger Him. And if we don't? Well, maybe He won't help.

But biblical scholars believe this completely misunderstands the parable—its real point being if neighbors might

129

help us only for selfish reasons, how much *more* will our *un*selfish Father help us.[1] We can therefore ask confidently (vv. 9–10), knowing God is greater than flawed human beings (vv. 11–13). God isn't the neighbor in the parable but the opposite of him.

Like it did for Richard, infertility can raise questions for us about God, prayer, and why tragic things like miscarriage happen. But to blame such tragedies on the way we have prayed both misunderstands God's goodness and unfairly burdens us.

"I don't know why you lost your baby," I told Richard. "But I know it wasn't because you didn't pray hard enough. Our God isn't like that."

Father, I bring my needs and the needs of others to You, confident You will hear and answer. I'm grateful it's Your goodness and not my words that count. You attend to each cry of my heart before I even utter it, and so I trust You today. Amen.

SHERIDAN VOYSEY

God doesn't need to be "badgered" to act. Ask confidently, knowing you've been heard.

Fur Babies

66

"Look at the birds of the air; they do not sow or reap or store away in barns, and yet your heavenly Father feeds them. Are you not much more valuable than they?"

MATTHEW 6:25–34

Why don't you just adopt?" If you haven't already been asked this question, you will be soon, as it's one of the most common (and annoying) questions asked of those yet to have kids. Fortunately, I have a quick response. "I did. She's a lovely little girl who eats tuna and wakes me at five in the morning with her meowing."

Yes, I adopted a fur baby—a rescue cat named Portia. And she's been a gift from God ever since.

I've read online criticisms of fur parents like me. Some think we must be desperate, or sad, or that we're "crazy cat ladies" (guilty as charged on that last one). But seriously, my fur baby makes me laugh when I'm sad, she gives me cuddles when I'm cold, and the sensation of her purring on my lap does something warm and fuzzy to my heart. She has made a difference in my life by helping me through the difficulties of growing our little family. Frankly, Portia has been a godsend.

In Matthew 6, Jesus told us our Father cares for us just as He cares for the birds of the air and flowers of the field

(vv. 26–30)—He wants to meet our needs well. When we crave comfort and connection, we can ask God to provide, knowing He will. He may provide connection through friends. He'll definitely provide comfort through His Holy Spirit, our companion in every situation (John 14:15–18). And He may even gift us with a fur baby to provide cuddles and laughter along the way.

Our Father wants to meet our needs. Let's bring those needs to Him and trust Him to meet them in fun, original, and creative ways.

Father, when I feel lonely, please provide comforters for me: the Holy Spirit, friends, even fur babies! When I am empty, please fill the void in my life. Show me You are present in every difficult moment. Thank You that You see my needs and are a good Father who provides for me. Amen.

STEPH PENNY

Don't overlook God's gifts of comfort and joy, including pets.

Follow the Leader

67

Trust in the LORD with all your heart
and lean not on your own understanding;
in all your ways submit to him,
and he will make your paths straight.

PROVERBS 3:5–6

Have you ever been confused by something in the Bible? It happens to me more often than I'd care to admit. Some things seem puzzling, others contradictory. How do I make sense of two seemingly conflicting truths?

For instance, I don't understand when God tells us to "be fruitful and increase in number" (Genesis 1:28), and yet that's the one thing I can't do. Why would He give a command like that and not enable me to carry it out? That's a hard truth for me to reconcile, and sometimes I wonder if His promises apply to others but not to me.

Then I read in Acts 1:8 where Jesus told us to be His witnesses in the world. And yet Paul and his companions were prevented from doing just that in the province of Asia (Acts 16:6). And again, when trying to enter Bithynia, "the Spirit of Jesus would not allow them to" (v. 7). They were so eager to spread the good news. Why prevent them from carrying out His command?

Praying Through Infertility

Infertility brings its fair share of obstacles. I think I know which direction to go but find I'm only forcing my way down another dead end. However, I'm learning these are really opportunities to submit my ways to Him and follow His alternative pathways. When I learn to trust where God is leading me, my crooked paths begin to look a whole lot straighter, even if I don't understand yet why I need to walk them (Proverbs 3:5–6).

Lord Jesus, I want to be obedient to Your commands even when it feels like I'm unable to carry them out. Let me not be discouraged but look for the ways You are leading me today. Give me patience and wisdom to understand Your direction for my life, even if it's not the direction I want to go or think I should be going. Amen.

NICHOLAS RICHARDSON

Could a roadblock be God's means of redirecting you down a different pathway?

Opting for Joy

—— 68 ——

Though the fig tree does not bud . . .
though there are no sheep in the pen . . .
yet I will rejoice in the LORD,
I will be joyful in God my Savior.

HABAKKUK 3:17–18

W e're pregnant!"

My heart still winces when friends utter these words. At times it's been hard to control my response to these happy people, and preferable to withdraw from them, lonely though it is. How my heart has desired to be joyful for my sisters and friends and their special news. Truly it wants to be, but my envy instead can urge me to buy a box of plates and smash them to smithereens!

Disappointment and devastation can hold a heart hostage, making it difficult to encounter joy. Habakkuk desperately sought God for answers to the problems of his people. He spoke candidly about his sorrow for the Jews, pleading with God for life to change. Yet despite life's dire landscape, he could still rejoice in the Lord: "Though the fig tree does not bud . . . though there are no sheep in the pen . . . I will rejoice in the LORD, I will be joyful in God my Savior" (Habakkuk 3:17– 18). Choosing this joy no doubt gave Habakkuk the resilience needed to endure the difficulties before him and find hope for a better future.

I frequently cling to these verses when I feel envy or disappointment arise. They are my lifeboat of hope, the balm for my wounds. Bringing this ancient lament into my own experience, I even add my own line to the passage: *Though there is no baby in my womb, I will rejoice in the Lord; I will be joyful in God my Savior.*

Opting for joy each day, connecting with God as our joy and delight (Psalm 43:4), has the power to stop envy from taking root, protect our hearts from anger and bitterness, and lead us to resilience and hope.

> *Dear God, I invite Your Holy Spirit to guard my heart and mind from the weight of my disappointment. Defend me from the clutches of despair that threaten to undermine my ability to be glad for others. Help me each day to dwell in Your sanctuary, choose joy, and find stability and restoration. Amen.*
>
> AMANDA PICKERING

Though there is no baby in my life, I will rejoice in the Lord; I will be joyful in God my Savior.

Suffering Is Part
of the Story

—————— 69 ——————

God is the one who began this good work in you,
and I am certain that he won't stop before it is
complete on the day that Christ Jesus returns.

PHILIPPIANS 1:3–6 CEV

The stories of infertility in Scripture used to frustrate me because they always ended with a baby. But when I looked closer, I noticed something. In each case Scripture gives more time to the struggle of infertility and unanswered prayer than the parenthood that follows.

For example, there are more verses dedicated to Hannah's anguish than her rejoicing when her son, Samuel, is finally born (1 Samuel 1; 2:1–10). Sarah's struggle to trust God's promise for a child spans a whole nineteen chapters in Genesis, but her story ends just two chapters after Isaac's birth. In each case, Scripture focuses on how God is deeply interested in each woman's mess and works in it.

This was transformative for me because I spent years fighting the pain caused by my infertility, believing it was getting in the way of the "good work" God wanted to do in my life (Philippians 1:6). But any good work God had started in these women's lives wasn't interrupted by their infertility but was *accelerated* by it. It was in their struggles that God was doing His best work in them—enlarging their stories, giving them eternal value. Hannah didn't just become a mother but the mother of Israel's first prophet (Acts 3:24; 13:20). And Sarah entered the lineage of Jesus (Matthew 1:2).

In a world where a good life is marketed as an effortless one, struggle has no home. But what I have grown to love about Scripture is how it consistently embraces suffering, reminding me that I'm not alone in mine, showing me God is ready to work in and through it for His kingdom and my good.

> *God of the brokenhearted, I thank You that You have always searched for the weak to fulfill Your purposes. You see my wounded heart and my fear of a future I never wanted. I invite You into this place of pain and ask that You begin a deeper work of transformation in me. Birth in me a bigger vision for this life and the life to come. Amen.*
>
> LIZZIE LOWRIE

God does His best work in us through times of suffering.

Pearls of Wisdom

————— 70 —————

Then you will live a life that honors the Lord,
and you will always please him. . . . His glorious
power will make you patient and strong enough to
endure anything, and you will be truly happy.

COLOSSIANS 1:10–11 CEV

They weren't kidding when they named it a waiting room. Like many others experiencing infertility, I spent countless hours in these rooms *waiting*. Waiting for tests. Waiting for results. Waiting to hear I was pregnant. As someone who values being productive, it felt like such a waste of my time— not only the hours the doctors kept me waiting, but the years God kept me in His waiting room as well. Since I had no one else to talk to in those silent rooms, I decided to spend that time talking to Jesus about this very thing.

One day in particular—a day I felt convinced I would never have the joy of pregnancy—I sensed Jesus give me a picture. It was of a strand of pearls around my neck, larger and more lustrous than I'd ever seen. The message was clear to me in an instant: Pearls are beautiful things born slowly out of irritation and persistence. Oysters do it by default, but with His help, I, too, could patiently persist and find something precious on the other side of my waiting.

I knew that vision of pearls wasn't a promise to fulfill my hopes for a child, but it was a promise of hope—that as I pursued a deeper connection with God through this trial, there *would* be positive results. As I trusted Him more, He would make me "strong enough to endure anything," as the apostle Paul said, making me "truly happy," beyond my circumstances (Colossians 1:10–11).

God wastes nothing. In His hands, whatever we are enduring today has the potential to shape our lives into ones that bring Him honor and us joy.

Lord, when I am waiting for answers or action, it can be easy to forget You are always working behind the scenes for my good. Help me to release my desire to control the outcome and instead trust Your plans for my future, knowing that You are a good Father and I am Your precious child.

LORI ALCORN

In our waiting and through our irritation,
God is creating something beautiful.

In Spite of, Not
Because Of

71

*Husbands, love your wives, just as Christ loved
the church and gave himself up for her.*
EPHESIANS 5:21–33

I live in a culture that glorifies having children. While marriage is held in high regard in Zimbabwe and other African countries, dissolving one because of infertility is seen as forgivable, and having children with someone else can even be tolerated. The reason? We Africans hardly believe it's possible to be childless *and* happy.

Since it's common to think the biological cause of infertility is on the wife's side, some would say I should divorce my wife for another woman or seek children outside our wedlock. But according to the gospel, procreation is not the glue that binds husband and wife together. It is *love* that cements that union, making our marriage complete without children. We are to love each other "despite" our infertility, not "because of" anything we could give each other.

The beauty of Christian marriage is that it's based on mutual submission out of reverence for Christ (Ephesians 5:21). We don't love our spouse because of what we can get from them but in spite of what we can't. May your marriage hold strong today as you walk this path together, showing the world what commitment really looks like through trial.

Father in heaven, thank You for giving me my life partner and for the example of love You've given us. Please make my marriage exemplary to both believers and unbelievers alike, as we draw from the fountain of Your love and learn to love each other unconditionally. Amen.

SIKHUMBUZO DUBE

---

*Infertility is an opportunity to learn
Christlike love for each other.*

Who You Are

_____ 72 _____

I praise you because I am fearfully and wonderfully made;
your works are wonderful, I know that full well.

PSALM 139:13–16

Our wedding nearly didn't happen. In the midst of excitedly deliberating over whether to add a blender to the gift list and poring over possible Bible readings for the service, I noticed my stomach protruding a little more than desired. After various scans and checks, a tumor the size of a soccer ball was discovered, swiftly followed by a surgeon explaining that the operation I required would result in my inability to conceive.

Knowing how much my fiancé, Andy, longed to be a father, I left the consultant's room and told him I would call off our engagement. The words he spoke next have stayed with me to this day: "I'm not marrying you because of what you can give me. I'm marrying you because of who you are." In that moment I received fresh insight into how the Lord delights in me irrespective of what I contribute to the world.

So often the message we hear from the world is that our worth is based on what we do or achieve. Believing this flawed message can mean that an inability to "achieve" parenthood could feel like a diminishment of our worth. But God doesn't value us like that. Even before we take our first breath or utter our first word, we are a marvel in His eyes—one of His wonderful works of art (Psalm 139:14).

Maybe, without realizing it, you have linked your worth to your ability to become a parent. If so, remember: God doesn't love you for what you can give Him or contribute to the world but for who you are—His wonderfully made work of art.

Creator God, in the areas where I don't yet fully believe how precious I am to You, let me know Your deep love for me. In the places where I do not yet see myself as You do, may I believe that I am "fearfully and wonderfully made." In the places where I need reassurance that I am enough as I am, may Your truth about me reign.

MARIA RODRIGUES

You are loved by God just as you are.
Right now, without exception.

Bread in the Wilderness

73

*All at once an angel touched him
and said, "Get up and eat."*

1 KINGS 19:1–18

A successful prophet at the top of his game fled into the wilderness and prayed that he might die. Depression can happen to anyone. It happened to Elijah, and a few months after my infertility diagnosis, it happened to me.

I had been "brave facing" and "staying strong" for as long as I could, but when the tears came, they were a torrent. I froze at my desk until, like Elijah, I fled into the wilderness—running out my office door into the forest nearby. It was a while before I was able to work again.

Breakdowns are exhausting. After Elijah ran, he lay down to sleep (1 Kings 19:3–5). There an angel met him and provided fresh bread and water (v. 6). When I opened up to others about my own situation, I found "angels" that provided care too: cooking meals, staying at my bedside, and praying when I couldn't.

Infertility can be like a daily walk into the wilderness, with cycles of trying or treatment requiring vast reserves of strength. The angel visited Elijah more than once (v. 7), and only when he was strengthened by food did Elijah journey on

(v. 8). I needed to allow myself time to be restored between treatments, however I could.

God had more in store for Elijah, meeting Elijah on a mountain where His gentle whisper restored his soul and restarted his mission (vv. 11–16). In the depths of my depression, there were moments of gentle grace too; times I sensed God speaking.

So my prayer today is that Elijah's story may be yours when you, too, feel like fleeing into the wilderness. May God's angelic messengers provide for you there. May you give yourself time to be strengthened before moving on. And may God's gentle whisper restore your soul.

Dear God, when I am weak, be strong for me. When I am surrounded by darkness, shine Your light. When I lose my way, send Your angels to direct me. When I am weary, give me rest. When I know not how to pray, send friends to pray for me. When I am hungry, give me the Bread of Life—Jesus Christ, my Lord. Amen.

ELIS MATTHEWS

What do you need from God in your wilderness moment?

Warning Signs

74

*Fix your thoughts on what is true, and honorable,
and right, and pure, and lovely, and admirable.
Think about things that are excellent and worthy of
praise. . . . Then the God of peace will be with you.*

PHILIPPIANS 4:8–9 NLT

When the engine light comes on in your car, do you ignore it or do you take it in and get it fixed? Our negative emotions can be a bit like that light—a gauge alerting us to trouble. I like to assess my level of irritability and anxiety on a scale from 1 to 10. If the number is high, I consider it a red-light indicator on my spiritual dashboard.

One day in the midst of our infertility journey, I decided to deal with the red-light warning signals I'd ignored for too long and take them to God. My time with God revealed the source of my anxiety—an upcoming fertility treatment—as well as a solution. I read that fixing my thoughts on what is true, lovely, and praiseworthy would lead to peace (Philippians 4:8–9). So I prayerfully set out to change the focus of my thoughts.

Instead of ruminating on the upcoming appointment, I made plans to go out for ice cream and a walk in the park afterward with my husband. It helped me to focus on the upcoming romantic time instead of the treatment. And instead of dwelling on the children I didn't have, I chose to think about what I did have—a warm house, a loving husband, caring parents. It made all the difference. My circumstances were the same, but I experienced contentment, peace, and even joy. Now when the warning lights come on, I am quicker to act and go to the Lord for His help.

Is irritability or anxiety getting the best of you? The Lord is ready to take a look at the problem and help you fix your thoughts on praiseworthy things—bringing the kind of peace that only He can give.

Lord Jesus, I come to You with my struggles. Your Word promises that Your yoke is easy and Your burden light (Matthew 11:30). Please take the weight of my anxieties and heal my heart. Help me to focus my thoughts on things that are lovely, noble, and true. On the days I struggle to see Your goodness, open my eyes to the beauty that surrounds me and fill me with Your peace. Amen.

JULIE RICHARDSON

What is true, lovely, and praiseworthy in your life and the world right now?

Joy Will Come

75

Weeping may last through the night,
but joy comes with the morning.

PSALM 30:1–5 NLT

Our first IVF cycle happened in 2003. Despite it not going smoothly (which is something of an understatement), the day came for two healthy-looking embryos to be transferred into my womb. One of those clusters of cells we saw on the screen might actually be our longed-for baby!

Then came the two-week wait before the pregnancy test. We were advised to go about life as usual—which was impossible, of course, with all our excitement and tangible hope at last. But just ten days later, I woke with a banging migraine and I started to bleed. It was all over. And it was Good Friday.

The irony of our loss happening on Good Friday didn't escape me, but I was too locked in devastation to make any real sense of the connection. In the days and months that followed, it felt like I got stuck, wondering if I'd ever get to the resurrection joy of Easter Sunday.

We can only imagine how the days between Jesus' death and His resurrection felt for the disciples. They must've felt shock, confusion, the raw pain of loss, and real fear for the future. Their best friend, their Master, was dead and buried. They didn't know of the joy to come.

Waiting is hard. Waiting without certainty is hardest. But when we struggle to see what God is doing, it doesn't mean He's not doing anything. "You brought me up from the grave, O Lord," David wrote. "Weeping may last through the night, but joy comes with the morning" (Psalm 30:3, 5 NLT). And just as Easter morning arrived for Jesus' disciples—bringing hope for the future—such a morning will arrive for us too. And with it, perhaps in unexpected places and unexpected ways, will come joy.

Heavenly Father, You know my hopes and dreams, my fears and struggles. And through Your Son, You know how it feels to be fearful and in pain. In my nights of weeping, may I feel Your love and comforting presence. Give me the strength to keep going, the assurance that You're walking the road with me, and the hope that I will again feel joy. Amen.

HANNAH SCOTT-JOYNT

Your joy will return.

Anthem

76

We have escaped like a bird
from the fowler's snare;
the snare has been broken,
and we have escaped.
Our help is in the name of the LORD,
the Maker of heaven and earth.

PSALM 124

Another negative pregnancy test, another shrug from a confounded doctor, another medication to try, and another attempt to get pregnant with all the fun and romance removed. Another year goes by, and then another, and another. More than a decade of this journey has strained our souls and stressed our marriage, yet somehow here we stand. Still together, still strong.

Reading Psalm 124 recently stirred something in my heart. In it I have found my anthem. My wife, Lizzie, and I had escaped the teeth of the "wild animals" and the flood that should've swept us away (vv. 3–6 CEV). The years of waiting should have crushed us; the endless invasive treatments should have broken our sanity; the ordeal should have ended our marriage. Yet, despite it all, we are not just standing but thriving. Our marriage is stronger, our faith is deeper, and our pain has been put to the service of others. None of this would have been our story "if the LORD had not been on our side" (v. 1).

It can be tempting to give up on faith, on marriage, on hope when going through this hardest of times. But persevere with God. He is on your side. And He is writing in you a new story, one worthy of its own anthem.

Father God, I thank You that today I'm still standing. I recommit myself to You afresh, placing my hope in Your faithfulness, asking that one day my own song might join with countless others that were rescued from the flood.

DAVID LOWRIE

God is on your side.

Faith in the Dark

77

By your words I can see where I'm going;
they throw a beam of light on my dark path.
PSALM 119:105–112 MSG

Before I went through infertility, I thought I had a firm grasp on what it meant to walk by faith. I thought I trusted God and His plans, whatever they would be. If we were blessed with children, we'd have the family we always wanted. If we weren't, I imagined us enjoying careers, holidays, and our disposable income. But when we got neither, I felt like I'd been dropped into a dark pit of nothingness, my thoughts filled with heartbreaking doubts that maybe God had forgotten me or didn't care. "I doubt Your control," I once told God in my prayer journal, "because I cannot see it."

Reflecting on that time now, I see that what I thought was "walking by faith" was in fact a misplaced confidence in my own envisaged plan. So when that plan didn't eventuate and all went dark, I had to *truly* trust God to move forward. Hard though it was, I soon realized this was really what walking by faith entailed—lifting my foot even if I had no idea where it would land, choosing to put my trust completely in something I knew to be true but couldn't see.

Maybe the way ahead looks dark for you now and you're

nervous about stepping forward. Faith in God isn't an easy choice, but it's never the wrong one. God gives us promises we can cling to in the dark—He'll never leave us to stumble (Psalm 37:23–24); His light cannot be extinguished (John 1:5); He'll provide a lamp for our feet and a light for our path (Psalm 119:105). Step forward in the dark confidently. Your steps are being guided by the Light of the World.

Jesus, take my hand. Thank You that You are always there. May I walk in Your light and trust Your vision, the One for whom dark and light are the same. If I could see the whole path, it would be too much for me, so I surrender it to You. Light my path and show me the blessings You've laid out for me along the way. Amen.

CLAIRE SANDYS

God doesn't want us to trust what we can see but what He can see.

Did God Close
My Womb?

78

The secret things belong to the LORD our God.

DEUTERONOMY 29:29

The fruitless scars of my surgeries are a constant reminder of the journey my husband and I have been on. Like a leaking roof on a rainy day, they sometimes drip damaging thoughts into my mind, making it moldy with negativity. One of the most persistent questions to bother me has been, *Did God close my womb?*

My infertility is considered by some in my culture to be punishment from God, like when friends of the patriarch Job thought the tragedy that befell him came because he'd sinned (Job 4:7–9). But when Job reviewed his life, he couldn't see any specific sins he might be punished for (13:23). Like him, I have wondered why God might have closed my womb when I'd done all the "right" things, like abstaining from sex until marriage. What was I being punished for?

Job never got answers to his questions on suffering, but *we* know his suffering wasn't due to any sin he'd committed (1:8–12). What Job did get was a revelation of God's character (chapters 38–42). That's where my question has led too. God is faithful and knows what is best in all situations. He is good and cannot be the source of evil. As someone has said, "God is too good to be unkind, too wise to be mistaken; and when you cannot trace His hand, you can trust His heart."[1]

Like Job and his suffering, I don't have clear answers as to why I don't have children. There are some answers God keeps to Himself (Deuteronomy 29:29). But I can confidently declare that "His mercy endures forever" (Psalm 136 NKJV).

Even when questions shake our spiritual foundation, "we will not fear, though the earth give way and the mountains fall into the heart of the sea" (Psalm 46:2). Because God is good, and we can trust Him.

Dear God, help me to trust in Your heart when I cannot trace Your hand. Help me to continually depend on You even when I'm in pain. Help me to wait on You so I can help those looking up to me. I trust in You today. Amen.

SONENI DUBE

You can trust God with your unanswered questions.

Relinquishing
the Questions

79

*"I know that you can do all things;
no purpose of yours can be thwarted."*

JOB 42:1–6

Merryn and I sat in church as the service ended. "Remember that thing Charlotte used to say when she didn't get her way?" she said, referring to how our niece, when she was two years old, used to tell her mother, "You're ruining me!" when she didn't get what she wanted. "In many ways," Merryn continued, "I've been saying the same thing to God about having a child: 'I *want* one. Why can't I *have* one? You're *ruining* me for not giving me one!' It's time for this to stop."

Merryn's words were significant. By this point we had tried for a decade to start a family, and her relationship with God had suffered as a result. But now she spoke peacefully, as one in whom a quiet breakthrough was happening.

There is a time to express our disappointment to God at His seeming lack of action in our situations. The psalmists repeatedly expressed such feelings (Psalm 13:1), as did prophets like Jeremiah (Jeremiah 20:7) and Habakkuk (Habakkuk 1:1–3). But like Job, there also comes a time to relinquish our questions to God, trusting His character when He doesn't give us answers (Job 42:1–3).

"I don't understand why God hasn't given us a child," Merryn said. "Perhaps I never will. But I know Him, and I know He wouldn't have meant this for evil." For just as there is a time to question, so there is a time to trust—allowing our *Why not?* to become a *What now?* in our relationship with God.

Lord, I ask You again today for a child, and give You my disappointment at not having one by now. I want to get to where Job got, realizing there are some things I may never understand, but trusting the outcome of this search to You, knowing You are utterly powerful, trustworthy, and good. In Jesus' name I pray, amen.

SHERIDAN VOYSEY

Is it time for your Why not? *to become a* What now?

The God Who Weeps

80

"Where have you laid him?" he asked.
"Come and see, Lord," they replied.
Jesus wept.

JOHN 11:32–36

As a child, I was struck by the story of Digory and Aslan in *The Magician's Nephew* by C. S. Lewis. The boy Digory hesitantly approaches Aslan to ask him to help his sick mother. When he finally plucks up the nerve to look Aslan in the face, he is astounded by what he sees: tears brimming in Aslan's majestic eyes. Aslan the lion weeps with Digory.[1]

When Jesus walked the earth He experienced sadness, disappointment, and grief. He was heartbroken over the fate about to befall Jerusalem (Luke 19:41–44). After sharing His need for support with His disciples in Gethsemane, they let Him down (Matthew 26:38–46). He wept at the tomb of his friend Lazarus (John 11:32–36). Jesus became fully human, joining with us in our suffering (Hebrews 2:5–9). Our God is a God who weeps.

One day I got angry with God, wondering why He was allowing the disappointment of infertility in my life. But in that moment I sensed a sudden closeness with Him—as if He were quietly sitting beside me, letting me cry. He didn't answer my questions. He didn't make me feel better. He just let me feel. And He felt my pain. Like Jesus at Lazarus's tomb, maybe He was even crying with me.

Psalm 34:18 says that God is close to the brokenhearted. When we feel sadness, when disappointment and grief arise, we can trust He is sitting there beside us. He will draw near and share in our pain, even through moments of sacred silence. When we are brokenhearted He is close at hand. And He weeps with us.

Father, when grief surfaces, please sit beside me and comfort me. Remind me that while You don't always heal pain, You always share in it. Be with me in the silence, in the weeping, in the sacred communion of grieving. Thank You for always hearing me, even when I don't speak a word. Amen.

STEPH PENNY

God sits with you in your pain and feels it.

Worship in the Wilderness

81

Water will gush forth in the wilderness
and streams in the desert.
ISAIAH 35:1–7

One of the hardest decisions Nick and I had to make was deciding when to stop fertility treatments. Our fear was that someday we would look back with regret. Might we have had a child if we'd kept going?

After seven years on the journey, Nick and I sensed the Lord calling us to stop our treatments. We left it in God's hands, stepping out in faith and hoping God would give us a child naturally. But after more years of waiting, my anticipation turned into a wilderness of disillusionment. I felt unseen and unheard by God. I felt forgotten.

Many years after that decision, I became a production assistant for the television program *Day of Discovery*, and I was soon on a plane to the Judean wilderness to film an episode with singer-songwriter Shannon Wexelberg, whose songs had been written out of her own struggle with infertility. As I listened to her sing out there in the desert, her lyrics gave expression to my own inner struggle and became a stream of life-giving water to me (Isaiah 35:6). Right there in the same wilderness where Jesus triumphed over Satan, I began to let go of my pain and inwardly worship God. And something happened—my soul was refreshed and my perspective changed. God's love enveloped me, and I realized He had been with me all along.

I am now in my fifties. Nick and I were never blessed with children, yet we have no regrets. While there has been grief, the intimacy of walking with Jesus has brought surprising joy along this path, giving it an unmatched beauty all its own.

Lord, thank You for Your living Word and promise to never leave us or forsake us. I know that Your Word is true in my head, but help me to experience it more deeply in my heart. Help me to see You at work in my life and to wholeheartedly worship You even in the wilderness. Amen.

JULIE RICHARDSON

Worship in your wilderness.

Wholehearted

82

The LORD is close to the brokenhearted
and saves those who are crushed in spirit.

PSALM 34:15–18

I felt my throat constrict against the impending tears. Heat flooded my face and I blinked rapidly to quell the onslaught. We had just stood to sing in our friends' large church, the words of the song jumping from the screen and taking my breath away.

The lyrics spoke of life breaking and dreams being taken away, but Jesus remaining our risen Lord, the One our hope comes from. I desperately wanted to sing this song, but tears streamed down my face instead. So I quietly stood there, whispering the words in my heart, my own dreams having been stripped away. I usually avoided crying in worship, doing everything in my power not to show my hurt. But this moment marked a shift in my relationship with God.

"The LORD is close to the brokenhearted and saves those who are crushed in spirit" (Psalm 34:18). As the psalmist reminded us, bringing our broken heart before God is a natural part of worship. In fact, the Bible is full of references and examples of being authentic with God (Lamentations 1:20; Psalm 25:17). After that day in church, no longer would I shamefully wipe away my tears, trying to disguise the salty healing balm that fell. My tears would now be an act of worship.

Infertility can make it hard to worship God with our whole selves. Be encouraged: God loves your broken heart, and bringing it with you into worship will only draw you closer to Him. Come as you are, and when words fail you, let your silence, your groans of lament, and your tears be your worship.

Lord, I want to worship You, but it's hard sometimes. May my broken heart and tears be acceptable to You on those days when they are all I have to give. Amen.

SHEILA MATTHEWS

Bring your whole self to God in worship, your tears and silences becoming an offering themselves.

Call Me Father

83

*See what great love the Father has lavished
on us, that we should be called children
of God! And that is what we are!*

1 JOHN 2:28–3:3

Who am I, then? The question haunted Francisco and me both for months. When we walked into the Young Marrieds Sunday school class at our church each Sunday, we'd see glowing pregnant women and content men holding children in their arms. That was supposed to be our identity too— Francisco a father, me a mother. Yet it wasn't. *Who are we, then?* we wondered.

The apostle John once penned a beautiful truth to a group of believers he cared deeply about. Written with passion, it's almost as if he took a deep breath, lifted his eyes to heaven, then exclaimed, "See what great love the Father has lavished on us, that we should be called children of God!" To make sure the message took hold, he added, "And that is what we are!" (1 John 3:1). Before being a father and a mother, before being anything or anyone else, we have this unlosable identity, knowing "all who do what is right are God's children" (2:29 NLT).

While Francisco and I later became parents, we didn't find

answers to all our questions during our infertility journey. But right in the middle of it, we did find Abba Father reassuring us that we were His children and that nothing, not even infertility, could separate us from that identity or from His love.

In times of wrestling with unfulfilled identities, each of us can rest in this: while we may not yet be a father or mother, we will always be our Father's child. And He loves us.

Abba Father, You know how much I long to hear a child's voice calling me "Father" or "Mother." Help me to rest in Your love and quiet myself enough to hear Your voice calling me "My child." Please give me the strength and will to walk in this identity every step of this difficult journey. In Jesus' name I pray, amen.

ESTERA PIROSCA ESCOBAR

Since Abba Father calls you His child,
you are loved and complete.

Victory over Resentment

84

Love is patient and kind; love does not envy or
boast; it is not arrogant or rude. It does not insist
on its own way; it is not irritable or resentful;
it does not rejoice at wrongdoing, but rejoices
with the truth. Love bears all things, believes all
things, hopes all things, endures all things.

1 Corinthians 13:4–7 ESV

As with many couples who've endured infertility, Lisa and I had moments of weakness along the path and, when we weren't careful, resentment entered our marriage. As pregnancies continued to fail, resentment toward each other grew—a toxic, cancerous thing for any relationship.

It isn't hard to feel angry or lose patience with each other during infertility, as our emotional stores are so often drained. Each partner may cope with infertility differently, perhaps needing more time alone than the other. Our personality differences come to the fore, which can be triggers for resentment too. There's no sugarcoating how difficult this can be, but I've learned the adversity of infertility can be withstood when both partners fight for their marriage by focusing on the love at the center of it.

The apostle Paul told us that love is patient and kind; it isn't irritable or resentful (1 Corinthians 13:4–5). What helped me to cultivate this kind of love for Lisa was remembering why I had married her in the first place. I wrote her notes recalling the love and attraction that originally brought us together and prioritized spending intentional time with her, knowing this was vital to expressing my love to her. My bride is my partner, and together in love we can bear all things— including any resentment arising during infertility.

The journey of infertility can be so tough, but I'm strengthened knowing I have Lisa through it and that she has me. Let's fight today for the love at the center of our marriages.

> Lord Jesus, help me to honor my spouse through all our difficulties. In times of weakness and resentment, remind me of our marriage covenant. May we bring each other closer to You and rejoice in the gift of our marriage. May we seek out each other's love and work to grow our relationship every moment. Amen.
>
> THOMAS NEWTON

Remind yourself of your love for each other every single day.

Heavenly Spouse

85

*"Do not be afraid; you will not be
put to shame. . . .
For your Maker is your husband—
the LORD Almighty is his name."*

ISAIAH 54:4–5

I didn't know my story was already in print until someone
recommended I read Isaiah 54. "That's me to a tee!" I said.
Here was a woman who had never borne a child (v. 1); who
felt afraid, ashamed, and humiliated (v. 4); who was deserted
and distressed in spirit (v. 6); and felt afflicted and lashed by
storms (v. 11). These verses made me feel understood for the
first time. I read them again and again.

The hero of this story quickly became my hero. He saw
me, moved toward me, and offered me what I yearned for—a
relationship of never-ending compassion, kindness, and love
(vv. 8, 10). This heavenly husband's credentials are awesome.
As my Maker, He understands me through and through
(v. 5)—how my body works, my fragility, my emotions. As
the Lord Almighty, He has full capability to meet my needs
and carry me through my struggles. As the Holy One of
Israel, His motives are pure and right, and as my Redeemer,

His life's work is to restore everything broken, bearing the cost Himself.

I love my husband, Tim. Infertility has tested our marriage in so many ways, yet we are stronger for it. But no earthly spouse can fulfill our deepest spiritual needs—only a heavenly spouse can do that. In Isaiah 54 I discovered that a heavenly spouse is the One who takes away the fear and shame of this infertility journey by His everlasting commitment to love us forever.

Heavenly Father, without You I would be crushed by feelings of fear, shame, and brokenness. Thank You for moving into my world with the offer of an intimate relationship and everlasting union so beautiful and hopeful that my negative experiences are displaced and replaced. I love You and trust You with my story. Amen.

DORCAS BERRY

Only God is a perfect spouse.

The Radar

86

*We know that in all things God works for
the good of those who love him, who have
been called according to his purpose.*

ROMANS 8:28–30

Church wasn't an easy place to be during our fertility treatments. There were too many lovely families with lovely kids, too many songs and points in the service that touched a nerve and left me in pieces. Some Sundays we'd spot a family getting out of their car, arriving for a christening, and turn around and drive home, unable to face another joyful service welcoming another child into the church family. (Our compassionate vicar started phoning us with "christening warnings"—pastoral care at its best.)

Several years on, we somehow had Charlie, who was welcomed into the church family with huge joy. But soon we noticed another couple who seemed to struggle with the same parts of the service and songs that we had and who were never at church for christenings. I asked the vicar if they were going through what we'd been through, and if so, to put us in touch. They were, he did, and the following week we were having coffee and talking fertility treatment with them.

Praying Through Infertility

That couple wasn't the only couple we sensed was secretly going through fertility troubles. Our experience seems to have given us a radar enabling us to spot them. And the stories shared and friendships forged as a result have been a huge gift to us all, as have the two precious goddaughters we've gained.

While I'm uneasy with the theology that God deliberately puts us through difficult things, what I do know is that He's used our tough stuff to help others through theirs—somehow redeeming our pain, enabling us to be a light along others' paths, working for their good.

Lord God, when life's a struggle and I'm in the middle of the tough stuff, I find it really difficult to see beyond it. But what a relief that You are the God of redemption and transformation, able to work in and through our experiences to bring light out of darkness, good things out of bad. Please open my eyes to the tough stuff in others' lives, that I might be Your light along their path. Amen.

HANNAH SCOTT-JOYNT

In the dark times, God is preparing you to be His light for others.

Dealing with Doubt

87

We are pressed . . . but we are not crushed. We are
perplexed, but not driven to despair. . . . We get
knocked down, but we are not destroyed.

2 CORINTHIANS 4:8–9 NLT

After a particularly difficult month, I flipped back through my journal. The feelings that jumped off its pages looked like they'd all camped out in the *D* section of the dictionary: I was depressed, discouraged, dismayed, and even doubtful of God's love. I had denied any idea of doubting God in the past, fearful He might reject me if I did. But now for the first time, the discouragement of my infertility was leading me to question whether God was as loving as I'd believed Him to be.

Struggling with this doubt and fear, I confided in a friend, who assured me my feelings didn't diminish God's love for me. After all, Jesus healed the son of a father who cried, "I believe; help my unbelief!" (Mark 9:24–25 ESV). My friend's advice was to keep my dialogue with God open and honest. As I did, God reminded me of the ways He'd faithfully loved me over the years, regardless of my faithfulness to Him. Like that doubting father, being honest about my doubts allowed God to guide me through them.

I also found help dealing with doubt from the apostle

Paul's words as he faced his own trials. When I was pressed by my troubles, I could press into God (2 Corinthians 4:8). When I was perplexed, I could turn to Him for truth. When I felt the knockdown punch of infertility, I could reach out for God to lift me back up again, continually turning to the One who never abandoned me (v. 9).

Like me, you may experience times when infertility leads you to doubt God's love for you. Start by being honest with Him. He will never leave you and longs to lead you through this.

Father God, I confess I sometimes find it hard to believe You are good when things don't unfold as I wish. I come to You with my doubts and ask that as I lean on You for understanding, You would help me see Your truth. Thank You for faithfully answering whenever I reach out to You, and for never letting anything come between us, not even myself.

LORI ALCORN

God can handle your honesty and even your doubt.

Wintering Moments

88

There is a time for everything,
and a season for every activity under the heavens.

ECCLESIASTES 3:1–14

I recently came across a helpful word: *wintering.* Just as winter is a time of slowing down in much of the natural world, author Katherine May uses this word to describe our need to rest and recuperate during life's "cold" seasons.[1] I found the analogy helpful after losing my father to cancer, which sapped me of energy for months. Resentful of this forced slowing down, I fought against my winter, praying that summer's life would return. I had much to learn.

Ecclesiastes famously says there's "a season for every activity under the heavens"—a time to plant and to harvest, to weep and to laugh, to mourn and to dance (3:1–4). I had read these words for years but only started to understand them in my wintering season. For though we have little control over them, each season is finite and will pass when its work is done. And while we can't always fathom what it is, God is doing something significant in us through them (v. 11). Just as plants and animals don't fight winter, I needed to rest and let it do its renewing work.

I wonder now how often I fought the wintering moments

of our infertility journey, trying to push through the energy-sapping experience of an adoption assessment or IVF round, when I really needed a season to recuperate.

"Lord," a friend prayed after I lost my father, "would You do Your good work in Sheridan during this difficult season?" It was a better prayer than my wish to rush back into summer's life. For in God's hands seasons are purposeful things and will pass when their work is done. Let's make space for such times of wintering, receiving His renewing work in each one.

Lord, You have something to do in me during this season of infertility. Thank You for using every season for Your glory and our good.

SHERIDAN VOYSEY

God is doing something important in your winter season. Make space to receive it.

The "Play-List"

89

There is a time for everything . . .
a time to mourn and a time to dance.
ECCLESIASTES 3:1–4

I have a keen interest in the field of positive psychology and often smile when I read research papers that confirm biblical wisdom. I recently read an article in which psychologist Dr. Barbara Fredrickson said, "All emotions—whether positive or negative—are adaptive in the right circumstances. The key seems to be finding a balance between the two."[1] In other words, there's an appropriate time to express each kind of emotion—essentially agreeing with Ecclesiastes that there's a right time to express joy and a right time to grieve (3:1–4).

As well as knowing it's okay to cry and lament when we walk through challenging times, it's also crucially important to find ways to have fun. Our son, Charlie, has his own Spotify playlist, an eclectic mix of music including everything from AC/DC and Ed Sheeran to Rend Collective. Whenever we put it on, it never fails to make us laugh as we dance and sing along. Like Charlie's music playlist, we need our own "play-list" of activities as a couple that enable us to experience joy, wonder, connection, and love. When Jon and I put our own list together, watching live sports, traveling, and having fun with friends were the first activities to be added.

Pete Greig, the founder of 24–7 Prayer, has said, "Suffering is inevitable in life, but joy is not. Pursue joy." He is so right. Unlike with pain and sadness, which life inevitably brings our way, we must be intentional when it comes to experiencing emotions like joy.

So what will be on your play-list of joyful activities? Once you create it, make sure to make time for these revitalizing pursuits.

Heavenly Father, thank You that there's a time for everything—including a time to laugh and dance. Please help us to intentionally create time and space for fun, laughter, and joy. Help us experience the truth that Your joy is our strength (Nehemiah 8:10). Amen.

KATHERINE GANTLETT

What activities will you include in your play-list?

The End of the Story

90

"He will wipe every tear from their eyes. There will be no more death" or mourning or crying or pain, for the old order of things has passed away.

REVELATION 21:1–7

The longing for motherhood and fatherhood can be breathtakingly difficult as we wrestle through our deferred dreams. Infertility is one of the oldest and most familiar struggles in history, and an often invisible and lonely journey. I know this longing, too, because I was born with a body that cannot bear babies.

In Genesis, we were called to be fruitful and multiply, but sin marred the world, including the ability for some to enter easily into natural parenthood. Our longings are a reminder that the world isn't as it should be. But for Christians, our earthly longings can point us to a deeper and truer reality.

When we cry, *How long, Lord?*, God meets us with the promise of Revelation 21. There He guaranteed that a day is coming when there will be no more death, mourning, or pain, when He will wipe every tear from our eyes (Revelation 21:4). Christian, we know the end of our story, and it is good.

How do we live this truth, though, on this side of eternity, neither dismissing our longings nor allowing them to consume us? We can make it our regular practice to bring our longings before the Lord, confident that He knows all about them (Psalm 38:9), that He promises His presence in the midst of them, and that those He doesn't fulfill now will be truly fulfilled in time.

A glorious day is coming when all will be redeemed and everything made right. Until that day, we can stake our hope in God's eternal, steadfast love. He is with us, right to the very end.

Father, only You truly know the depth of our longing. We trust You with it, even when grief and sorrow are our constant companions. Give us eyes to see Your goodness and faithfulness each day and train us to trust in Your promises as we bring these longings to You. Thank You for walking this path with us to the very end. Amen.

CHELSEA SOBOLIK

Let your earthly longings point you to the perfect fulfillment of eternity. To download a Couples Discussion Guide for this book, and for more help and resources, please visit:

www.prayingthroughinfertility.com

Acknowledgments

Compiling *Praying Through Infertility* has been a special experience. To bring such a variety of contributors together, both men and women, from so many countries, on such a sensitive topic, feels incredibly important. Many who've shared their stories in these pages did so for the first time, and I'm grateful for the courage, vulnerability, and insights they've shared. To each of my fellow writers—know that your words have gifted us with companionship, wisdom, and encouragement that couldn't have come from anyone else. Thank you.

It's a gift to have allies on this journey. Stephanie Newton, associate publisher at W Publishing, has been one of them. I first met Stephanie through writing *Resurrection Year*, a book she cheered on more than anyone. *Praying Through Infertility* was Stephanie's idea, and at first, with other projects on, I wasn't sure it was mine to do. But when I realized this could be a collaborative book, written with fellow travelers that *Resurrection Year* had helped me meet, a light switched on. Stephanie, the interest you've shown this community by

Acknowledgments

championing projects like this has helped link us together and bring hope to many.

I'm grateful, too, for a small group of people whose early feedback helped confirm and sharpen the book's content. Thank you, Angela Bonnici, Emily Ch'ng, Michael and Sofia Chu, Luke Denley, Jelvin and Vanessa Lee, Emily Pignon, and Vilborg Zielke for your vital input. And thank you to my wife, Merryn Voysey, for being willing to have our own story go "out there" again and for her helpful advice on the book's final form.

Finally, thank you to the team at W Publishing. From editorial to design to marketing to sales, I'm grateful your passion to inspire the world through good books comes with an equal commitment to faith and excellence.

Notes

Introduction: You Are Not Alone

1. "Cristo degli Abissi (Christ of the Abyss)," Atlas Obscura, May 20, 2013, https://www.atlasobscura.com/places/christ-of-the-abyss-italy.

Chapter 27: Beat Again

1. "Phillips, Craig & Dean—'Tell Your Heart to Beat Again' Story Behind the Song," Fair Trade Services, YouTube, May 9, 2012, https://www.youtube.com/watch?v=pdPp7ofeBMA.

Chapter 30: Think About Your Thinking

1. Julie Tseng and Jordan Poppenk, "Brain Meta-State Transitions Demarcate Thoughts Across Task Contexts Exposing the Mental Noise of Trait Neuroticism," *Nature Communications* 11 (July 2020), https://doi.org/10.1038/s41467-020-17255-9.

2. Stephanie Bogan, "Silence Those Voices in Your Head," Investment News, November 30, 2016, https://www.investmentnews.com/silence-those-voices-in-your-head-69986.

Chapter 37: Training for Triumph

1. John S. Mbiti, *African Religions and Philosophy* (London: Heineman, 1969), 107.

Notes

Chapter 38: My Best Friend

1. Albert Midlane, "There's a Friend for Little Children," 1859, Golden Bells Hymnal (London: Scripture Union, 1925). Public domain.
2. Midlane, "There's a Friend for Little Children."

Chapter 41: Learning to Lament

1. Matt Lynch, "A Time for Minor Chords: The Costly Loss of Lament in Contemporary Worship," *Theological Miscellany* (blog), WTC Theology, February 28, 2017, https://wtctheology .org.uk/theomisc/time-minor-chords-costly-loss-lament -contemporary-worship/.

Chapter 42: Five Good Things

1. Jason Marsh, "Tips for Keeping a Gratitude Journal," *Greater Good Magazine*, University of California, Berkeley, November 17, 2011, https://greatergood.berkeley.edu/article/item/tips_for_keeping _a_gratitude_journal.

Chapter 43: Finding Contentment

1. Johnson Oatman, "Count Your Blessings," public domain, https:// hymnary.org/text/when_upon_lifes_billows_you_are_tempest.

Chapter 51: A Seat at the Table

1. Richard Rohr, *The Divine Dance* (London: SPCK, 2016), 30–31.

Chapter 52: Moments of Reprieve

1. "Don't Stop Me Now," track 12 on Queen, *Jazz*, Super Bear Studios, 1978.

Chapter 57: Faith Through the Fire

1. Bill Johnson, *Strengthen Yourself in the Lord Study Guide* (Shippensburg, PA: Destiny Image Publishers, 2007), 153.

Chapter 59: Bottle of Tears

1. J. Alasdair Groves and Winston T. Smith, *Untangling Emotions* (Wheaton, IL: Crossway, 2019), chapter 17.

Notes

Chapter 65: Not Like That

1. Klyne Snodgrass, *Stories with Intent: A Comprehensive Guide to the Parables of Jesus* (Grand Rapids, MI: Eerdmans, 2018), 441–48.

Chapter 78: Did God Close My Womb?

1. Although this beautiful quote is often attributed to Charles Spurgeon, its originator is unknown.

Chapter 80: The God Who Weeps

1. C.S. Lewis, *The Magician's Nephew* (London: The Bodley Head, 1955), chapter 12.

Chapter 88: Wintering Moments

1. Katherine May, *Wintering: The Power of Rest and Retreat in Difficult Times* (New York: Riverhead Books, 2020).

Chapter 89: The "Play-List"

1. "Positive Emotions and Your Health: Developing a Brighter Outlook," *NIH News in Health*, August 2015, https://newsinhealth.nih.gov/2015/08/positive-emotions-your-health.

About the Contributors

Lori Alcorn is an author and infertility coach, empowering women experiencing detours to motherhood. She is the author of *The Pregnant Pause*, which shares her story of infertility and her journey to finding joy again. Lori has been married to Sean since 2003, and they recently downsized to country life just outside of Winnipeg, Canada. Lori can be found at **www.atalossinfertility.com**.

Dorcas Berry has taught modern languages and served in local church ministry alongside her husband, Tim. Her life, work, and her own struggle with infertility has been massively helped by studying biblical counseling, a field she loves. After several years on the island of Guernsey off the French coast, Dorcas and Tim have recently returned to the United Kingdom.

Tim Berry is a pastor and evangelist, most recently serving on the island of Guernsey, and before that in Derbyshire, United Kingdom. He has a passion for helping fellow saints, sufferers, and sinners through biblical counseling. Tim and his wife, Dorcas, currently live in North Devon awaiting their next ministry opportunity.

Giulianna Corrêa has a degree in mechanical engineering and works in the oil and gas industry. In addition to her job as an engineer, she loves to serve God through worship ministry. Giulianna lives in Brazil with her husband, Rômulo; daughter, Laura; and their dog, Dory. She loves to travel and discover new cultures.

Rômulo Corrêa is a businessman and pastor, serving in pastoral ministry to youth for over ten years. Rômulo is married to Giulianna, and their daughter, Laura, is their beautiful miracle. Rômulo and his family live in Curitiba, in southern Brazil, and he travels the world preaching Christ.

Sikhumbuzo Dube is an ordained Seventh-day Adventist pastor, a health-care chaplain, and a church administrator. He has published several articles on spiritual care, chaplaincy, and involuntary childlessness. Sikhumbuzo is the founder of Shunem Care, a ministry to involuntarily childless people. He is married to Soneni, and they live in Bulawayo, Zimbabwe. **www.shunemcare.home.blog**

Soneni Dube is an accountant holding a bachelor of business administration accounting degree from Solusi University and is currently pursuing a master's degree in business administration. She is married to Sikhumbuzo, and they live in Bulawayo, Zimbabwe. Her desire to see childless marriages thrive motivated her and her husband to start Shunem Care, a ministry to involuntarily childless people. **www.shunemcare.home.blog**

Estera Pirosca Escobar is an author, speaker, intercultural trainer, and sought-after Perspectives on the World Christian Movement instructor. Originally from Romania, Estera is married to Francisco, a global nomad originally from Chile. After a season of miscarriages and infertility, they were blessed with a beautiful daughter, Esmeralda. Together they enjoy welcoming internationals to their home in Nashville, Tennessee.

Edwin Estioko is a Philippines-based writer and illustrator of children's books and early childhood educational materials. He serves as senior photojournalist for Compassion International, a global child-sponsorship organization. Edwin is married to Daisy, and they live with their three beautiful children in the capital city of Manila. Since the pandemic their family has adopted three dogs, four cats, and two rabbits.

Justine Froelker has been a licensed professional counselor for over twenty years and certified in the work of Dr. Brené Brown since 2014. She has authored nine books, including five

About the Contributors

Amazon bestsellers, and speaks globally on leadership and courageous resilience. Justine lives in St. Louis, Missouri, with her husband, Chad; their three dogs; and during each summer, hundreds of monarch butterflies.
www.justinefroelker.com

Katherine Gantlett studied theology at Westminster Theological Centre and lives in rural Oxfordshire in the United Kingdom, with her son and husband. She has a background in biomedical science with a PhD from the University of Oxford in HIV research. Katherine is the author of *Walking Through Winter*, which explores how we can walk through seasons of loss with authenticity, faith, and hope.
www.katherinegantlett.org.uk

Jenn Hesse is the coauthor of *Waiting in Hope: 31 Reflections for Walking with God Through Infertility*. She is the content director of Waiting in Hope Ministries and a freelance writer contributing to Christian media outlets. Jenn and her husband, Colin, and their three sons live in Oregon, and cheer for the Seattle Seahawks, rain or shine.
www.jennhesse.com

Sarah Lang cofounded The Rhythm of Hope ministry with her husband, Andy. They live in a thatched cottage in the Oxfordshire countryside of the United Kingdom. Sarah is a pediatric nurse and has been involved in church leadership,

worship, preaching, and radio. Sarah often surprises people with her love of boxing (both watching and doing!) and her ability to instantly say words backward.
www.therhythmofhope.co.uk

Angeline Leong is a parish worker at My Saviour's Church, an Anglican church in Singapore. A graduate of Trinity Theological College, Singapore, she is passionate about teaching the Bible, seeing lives transformed, and helping families in need. Angeline is married to Louis, also in pastoral ministry, and they are blessed with two biological daughters and several godchildren.

David Lowrie is a pioneer minister in the Church of England and cofounder of StoryHouse, a coffee shop and church. He writes about his experience of childlessness as part of the Saltwater and Honey collective (**www.saltwaterandhoney.org**). David is married to the incredibly talented Lizzie and is loving life in Liverpool, United Kingdom.

Lizzie Lowrie is an author, speaker, and lay pioneer living in Liverpool with her husband, Dave, and their dog, Betsy. Lizzie writes about infertility, miscarriage, childlessness, and faith in her memoir, *Salt Water and Honey*, and on **www.saltwaterandhoney.org**. She is also the colead pastor of StoryHouse, an independent coffee shop and church she started with Dave.

About the Contributors

Elis Matthews is a vicar in the Church of England, responsible for two churches on the outskirts of London. A part-time poet with a heart for adventure, he walked the Camino de Santiago to celebrate his fortieth birthday. He was Spoken Word Artist in Residence for the charity All We Can and cofounded the *Saltwater and Honey* blog.

Sheila Matthews is a part-time educator, full-time dreamer, teacher turned writer, and proud Londoner. She is married to Elis, an Anglican vicar, and mother to Barney, a seven-year-old *Minecraft* aficionado who delights and exhausts his parents with gusto. Sheila also cofounded *Saltwater and Honey*, a blog and community for people experiencing infertility and childlessness: www.saltwaterandhoney.org.

Civilla M. Morgan is an author, blogger, and founder of the *Childless Not by Choice* podcast. She is passionate about writing and the spoken word. Civilla truly feels in her element when encouraging others to be all they can be. She does not have much time to relax, but she feels fortunate to live in Florida, where there are tons of beaches to choose from. www.civillamorgan.com

Lisa Newton is the author of *31 Days of Prayer During Infertility* and writes a popular blog encouraging women going through infertility. She works part-time as a children's story-time librarian, hates coffee but will never turn down a good cup of tea, and lives with her husband, Tom, and their two children near Monterey, California. **www.amateurnester.com**

Thomas Newton is a high school principal and has been an educator for seventeen years. He is an avid reader, sports enthusiast, and wine lover. His wife, Lisa, blogs about infertility at **www.amateurnester.com**. They have been married since 2011 and live with their two children near the beautiful coastal city of Monterey, California.

Steph Penny is the author of *Surviving Childlessness* and *Surviving Singledom*. She is a blogger, songwriter, musician, and lover of fur babies. In her spare time Steph works as a psychologist in the addiction field. When she's not working or writing, you can find Steph reading or indulging in her favorite chocolate dessert. **www.stephpenny.com.au**

Alex Pickering has loved the Lord since primary school. He was diagnosed with unexplained infertility and chose a path of no intervention, trusting the future to God. He loves music, snowboarding, kicking a football with his nephews and nieces, and playing Monopoly with friends. Married to Amanda, he is a marketing director living in Petersfield in the United Kingdom.

Amanda Pickering is married to Alex and enjoys cycling, dancing, friendship, and optimizing storage. Passionate about administration, her career has focused on executive assistant roles. Diagnosed with unexplained infertility in 2012, she opted not to pursue intervention but to embrace a life of acceptance, relying on Jesus as her faithful companion along the journey.

Rachel Quinlan is a full-time pharmacist and a licensed reader in the Church of England. She and her husband, Graham, live in Hertfordshire, United Kingdom, and they enjoy holidays and long walks in the countryside. Rachel is an avid reader and has recently taken up fitness challenges like the Couch to 5k running program.

Justin Ramsey is the cofounder of Waiting in Hope Ministries, a dentist, and an entrepreneur. He loves systems and business challenges as well as making people feel welcome and seen. Justin; his wife, Kelley; and their two boys live in The Woodlands, Texas, and are in the process of growing their family further through adoption. **www.waitinginhopeinfertility.com.**

Kelley Ramsey is the coauthor of *Waiting in Hope: 31 Reflections for Walking with God Through Infertility*. She is the founder and visionary of Waiting in Hope Ministries, and a speaker, teacher, and leader with a heart for discipleship. Kelley; her husband, Justin; and their two sons live in The Woodlands, Texas and are on another adventure as a waiting adoptive family. **www.waitinginhopeinfertility.com.**

About the Contributors

Julie Richardson is a visual media producer with Our Daily Bread Ministries. Her video productions have taken her all over the world, including Israel, Turkey, and Greece. Julie has led women's ministries in her local church and a variety of nonprofit ministries. She enjoys photography and, with her husband, Nick, has recently taken up sailing.

Nicholas Richardson is the senior graphic designer for Kregel Publications, where he has worked for nearly thirty years. In his local church he has served as a guitarist on the worship team and as an elder. He and his wife, Julie, love to hike, and they enjoy spending time with their families.

Maria Rodrigues hosts a daily live radio show across the United Kingdom. She has a master of arts in theology, teaches at conferences across the United Kingdom, and has served on the international leadership team for a Christian covenant community. Maria is married to Andy, and they love investing in upcoming generations through running youth groups, pilgrimages, and mission trips.

Pete Roscoe is married to Emma, a general practitioner, and a proud dad to three amazing children. He is a consultant in emergency medicine in northern England and author of *Man Up to Infertility*, which recounts Pete and Emma's journey through infertility and adoption. In his limited free time, Pete loves cycling and paddleboarding on the Welsh coast of the United Kingdom.

About the Contributors

Chris Sandys is a radio producer and podcaster. He has spent twenty years in local BBC radio and hosts *The Silent Why* podcast with his wife, Claire, about finding hope in loss. In 2010 he learned he was infertile due to surgery he'd had as a child. Chris and Claire live in Gloucestershire, United Kingdom, where Chris enjoys cycling, listening to music, and eating everything Claire bakes.
www.thesilentwhy.com

Claire Sandys is a writer, blogger, and host of *The Silent Why* podcast, where she explores themes of grief and loss inspired by her own experience of loss through childlessness. She has been married to Chris since 2005, and they live in beautiful Gloucestershire, United Kingdom, where she enjoys baking sweet treats and watching hedgehogs in the garden at night.
www.thesilentwhy.com

Hannah Scott-Joynt is a voiceover artist, broadcaster, producer, and ordinand for local ministry in the Church of England. She is married to Jonathan, a TV and radio producer, and they feel incredibly fortunate to have had their son, Charlie, after five years of fertility treatment. Hannah and her family live in Surrey, United Kingdom, with a daft Cavapoo called Ziggy.

Chelsea Sobolik is the author of *Longing for Motherhood: Holding On to Hope in the Midst of Childlessness* and a forthcoming book on women and work. She was adopted

About the Contributors

from Romania, grew up in North Carolina, and lives in Washington, DC, with her husband, Michael, where she works on public policy. **www.chelseapattersonsobolik.com**

Karen Swallow Prior and her husband, Roy, married young, and all these decades later wouldn't have had it any other way. Although they never had their own children, they are both teachers and are thankful for the ways they've been able to invest in the lives of so many childern over the years. They live on a few acres in rural Virginia, where Karen's parents, dogs, and several chickens also make their home. **www.karenswallowprior.com**

Sheridan Voysey is an author, speaker, and broadcaster, regularly contributing to BBC Radio 2 and other radio networks. He is the author of *Resurrection Year* and *The Making of Us*, which recount his and his wife's infertility story in detail. Sheridan is married to Merryn, a medical research professor at Oxford University, and they live in Oxford, United Kingdom, with their cheeky dog, Rupert. **www.sheridanvoysey.com**

About the Complier
and Contributor

Sheridan Voysey is an author, speaker, broadcaster, and founder of Friendship Lab. His other books include *Resurrection Year: Turning Broken Dreams into New Beginnings*, which recounts his and his wife's infertility story in detail, and *The Making of Us: Who We Can Become When Life Doesn't Go as Planned*.

Sheridan is a regular contributor to BBC Radio 2 and other international networks, has been featured on BBC Breakfast, BBC News, Day of Discovery, and CBC Canada's *Tapestry*, and in publications such as *The Times* and *The Sunday Telegraph*. He writes for the globally read devotional *Our Daily Bread*.

Sheridan is married to Merryn, a medical research professor at Oxford University, and they live in Oxford, United Kingdom, with their cheeky dog, Rupert.

For more information, visit www.sheridanvoysey.com or www.friendshiplab.org.

Perhaps a greater tragedy than a broken
dream is a life forever defined by it.

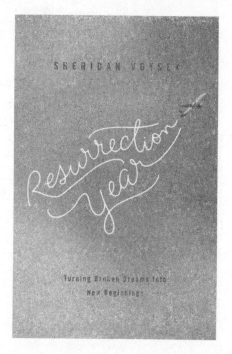

"Sheridan Voysey writes from experience—there is life after the
death of a dream. Your dream may be different, but the road to
resurrection will be similar. I highly recommend it."

—Gary Chapman, author of *The Five Love Languages*

"*Resurrection Year* is a gift that will breathe life and hope into
many who have faced a broken dream."

—Darlene Zschech

Beautiful things can emerge from life
not going to plan. It can even be . . .

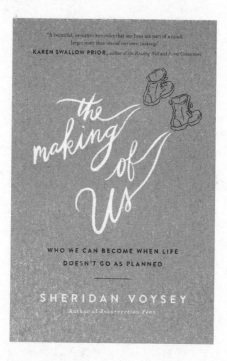

"A beautiful, evocative reminder that our lives are part of a much
larger story than oneof our own making."
KAREN SWALLOW PRIOR, author of On Reading Well and Love Correction

the
making
of
us

WHO WE CAN BECOME WHEN LIFE
DOESN'T GO AS PLANNED

SHERIDAN VOYSEY
Author of Resurrection Year

"A compelling trek that reveals how dissonance and
disruption can call us into the delight of God."
—Dan Allender

"An exceptional read."
—Adria Plass